CALLING FAMILY

MEDICAL ANTHROPOLOGY: HEALTH, INEQUALITY, AND SOCIAL JUSTICE

Series editor: Lenore Manderson

Books in the Medical Anthropology series are concerned with social patterns of and social responses to ill health, disease, and suffering, and how social exclusion and social justice shape health and healing outcomes. The series is designed to reflect the diversity of contemporary medical anthropological research and writing, and will offer scholars a forum to publish work that showcases the theoretical sophistication, methodological soundness, and ethnographic richness of the field.

Books in the series may include studies on the organization and movement of peoples, technologies, and treatments, how inequalities pattern access to these, and how individuals, communities, and states respond to various assaults on well-being, including from illness, disaster, and violence.

For a list of all the titles in the series, please see the last page of the book.

CALLING FAMILY

Digital Technologies and the
Making of Transnational
Care Collectives

TANJA AHLIN

RUTGERS UNIVERSITY PRESS
New Brunswick, Camden, and Newark, New Jersey
London and Oxford

Rutgers University Press is a department of Rutgers, The State University of New Jersey, one of the leading public research universities in the nation. By publishing worldwide, it furthers the University's mission of dedication to excellence in teaching, scholarship, research, and clinical care.

Library of Congress Cataloging-in-Publication Data

Names: Ahlin, Tanja, author.
Title: Calling family : digital technologies and the making of transnational care collectives / Tanja Ahlin.
Description: New Brunswick : Rutgers University Press, [2023] |
    Series: Medical anthropology: health, inequality, and social justice |
    Includes bibliographical references and index.
Identifiers: LCCN 2022054640 | ISBN 9781978834323 (paperback) |
    ISBN 9781978834330 (hardcover) | ISBN 9781978834347 (epub) |
    ISBN 9781978834354 (pdf)
Subjects: LCSH: Older people—Care—India. | Adult children of aging parents—India. | Familes—India—Psychological aspects.
Classification: LCC HV1484.I42 A37 2023 | DDC 362.60954—dc23/eng/20230302
LC record available at https://lccn.loc.gov/2022054640

A British Cataloging-in-Publication record for this book is available from the British Library.

rutgersuniversitypress.org

To my care collective across borders
mati, Mitja, Aria
ata pa mama

CONTENTS

FOREWORD

LENORE MANDERSON

The Medical Anthropology: Health, Inequality, and Social Justice series is concerned with the diversity of contemporary medical anthropological research and writing. The beauty of ethnography is its capacity, through storytelling, to make sense of suffering as a social experience and to set it in context. Central to our focus in this series, therefore, is the way in which social structures, political and economic systems, and ideologies shape the likelihood and impact of infections, injuries, bodily ruptures and disease, chronic conditions and disability, treatment and care, and social repair and death.

Health and illness are social facts; the circumstances of the maintenance and loss of health are always and everywhere shaped by structural, local, and global relations. Social formations and relations, culture, economy, and political organization as much as ecology shape experiences of illness, disability, and disadvantage. The authors of the monographs in this series are concerned centrally with health and illness, healing practices, and access to care, but in the different volumes the authors highlight the importance of such differences in context as expressed and experienced at individual, household, and wider levels. Health risks and outcomes of social structure and household economy (for example, health systems factors) as well as national and global politics and economics all shape people's lives. In their accounts of health, inequality, and social justice, the authors move across social circumstances, health conditions, geography, and their intersections and interactions to demonstrate how individuals, communities, and states manage assaults on people's health and well-being.

As medical anthropologists have long illustrated, the relationships between social context and health status are complex. In addressing these questions, the authors in this series showcase the theoretical sophistication, methodological rigor, and empirical richness of the field while expanding a map of illness, social interaction, and institutional life to illustrate the effects of material conditions and social meanings in troubling and surprising ways. The books reflect medical anthropology as a constantly changing field of scholarship, drawing on research in such diverse contexts as residential and virtual communities, clinics, laboratories, and emergency care and public health settings; with service providers, individual healers, and households; and with social bodies, human bodies, biologies, and biographies. Although medical anthropology once concentrated on systems of healing, particular diseases, and embodied experiences, today the field has expanded to include environmental disasters, war, science, technology, faith, gender-based violence, and forced migration. Curiosity about the body and its vicissitudes remains a pivot of our work, but our concerns are with the location of bodies in social life and with how social structures, temporal imperatives, and shifting exigencies shape life courses. This dynamic field reflects the ethics of the discipline to address these pressing issues of our time.

As the subtitle of the series indicates, the books center on social exclusion and inclusion, social justice and repair. The volumes in this series illustrate multiple ways in which globalization and national and local inequalities shape health experiences and outcomes across space; economic, political, and social inequalities influence the likelihood of poor health and its outcomes in different settings. At the same time, social and economic relations enable the institutionalization of poverty; they produce the unequal conditions of everyday life and work, and hence, also, of who gets sick and who is most likely to survive. The books challenge readers to reflect on suffering, deficit, and despair within families and communities while they also encourage readers to remain alert to resistance and restitution—to consider how people respond to injustices and evade the fissures that might seem to predetermine their lives.

The established laws of kinship and marriage, the conventions of locality, naming, and inheritance, and the relative roles and responsibilities of gender vary by age, lineage, and affinity, yet everywhere they determine the texture of everyday life. They determine the work undertaken within domestic and productive institutions, too, and they define the relationships that bind them and wrap around them. Kinship norms guide who provides what kinds of care within familial and wider social networks. Such care is first that delivered to children to ensure their safety, optimal development, and security. But such norms also guide where and how care takes place for other people, including those with developmental and functional challenges, and those who, with illness, injury, or aging, lose a measure of independence and require increasing support.

Economic and political changes over the past century have changed what is needed and expected in the provision of care, and it is no longer taken for granted that the youngest daughter (in one context) or the eldest son's wife (in another) will be at home, caring for aging parents or parents-in-law. In some settings where economic life is deeply troubled and unemployment is rife, including in much of rural South Africa, for instance, the care work has devolved to unemployed grandchildren and great-grandchildren regardless of gender. In other cases, people are left alone, excepting for occasional visits to neighbors, while children who might once have provided care send money as available from distant cities.

In many countries, overseas and interstate migration has disrupted predictable rhythms of care, how care is defined, and the pathways of its delivery. Worldwide, an estimated 281 million people are international immigrants, the majority of whom have moved in search of better economic opportunities. A significant proportion of these are health workers from all fields seeking better conditions and better pay in higher income countries, who are encouraged to move by host countries to meet their own workforce needs. Canada and the United States, Europe, Australia and New Zealand, and countries in the United Arab Emirates all recruit foreign-trained workers in face of national shortfalls of nurses and other care-related workers. Increasingly, professionalized and home-based care in wealthy countries is dependent on migration. These out-migrants leave shortfalls in their countries of origin in consequence, in the hospitals, health centers and institutions, and private family homes. For these workers are all the children of someone, and they are often the parents of others. In consequence, familial roles of care and residence have been disrupted, economic and interpersonal relationships between generations have been transformed, and new ways of care are being invented (Hromadžić and Palmberger 2018).

In *Calling Family: Digital Technologies and the Making of Transnational Care Collectives,* Tanja Ahlin describes the personal context of this flow from home to host country. In India, because they sit astride the constraints of Hindu caste rules and Moslem gender constraints, the majority of nurses are Christian. A significant number of these nurses are from the far southern state of Kerala, including from the Syrian Christian community. Among this population, young women (and men) are encouraged to train as and find employment as nurses; with additional English language skills, they have the option of recruitment into a global health workforce. From this standpoint, their remittances support their families in India—their aged parents, other siblings, spouses, parents-in-law, and children. The money they send is enough to pay for servants and childcare, school fees and medicines, better, grander, and more spacious houses and cars, and televisions and computers. Out-migration is the price of a contemporary, cash-dependent and materially enriched life. It is also a care practice.

But care does not only involve the flow of money and the purchase of goods and services. Depending on the availability of communication networks, the increased ownership and use of smartphones, computers, and notebooks and their various social media platforms—Facebook, Zoom, WhatsApp, and the like—have aided family members and health professionals to provide personalized forms of care and support older people to manage illness and frailty, regardless of location or distance (Prendergast and Garattini 2015; Cabalquinto 2022).

In *Calling Family,* Tanja Ahlin asks how out-migrant nurses provide care for older kin, mostly parents, at a distance and abroad. She illustrates how care is enacted with digital technology as an essential technology. The technology, the networks that support communication, the people who work these, the families and individuals in home and work settings in different countries, the times and activities that enable calls, the digital remittance of money, and the support, advice, and mundane exchanges of information—these transnational care collectives allow people to come together for practical and affective care work. Digital technologies allow nurses the means to review health problems at home.

The smartphone in particular allows nurses to see the problem, provide advice on self-care and medication, offer their interpretations and opinions of medical judgments, and facilitate and review referrals. It allows children to express sympathy to their parents, to listen to everyday complaints, and to reassure those for whom they care that they are available—they are only a phone call away. Technology allows for care to be enacted, even though mediated by distance and delivered by others (who are often paid wages themselves) in their parents' homes. As Tanja Ahlin illustrates, the regularity and frequency of calls—once, twice, or three times day—enable discussion of the questions of everyday life, the ways in which care and affection might be enacted were the caller and called in the same room. And these regular calls allow the conviviality that might otherwise be lost: the kind that occurs as people sit side by side viewing television, or eating a meal, or watching children play. Affect motivates the use of digital technology, and sim cards and Wi-Fi connections enable affective care.

As Tanja Ahlin illustrates through her rich ethnographic descriptions from homes both in Kerala and in Oman, care flows in all directions between individuals in families and for the technologies on which they rely. The nurses with whom she worked most closely live simply, ensuring that the money they set aside from their wages is adequate to remit to meet the costs of care at home so that their long sojourns make a difference. Often they are alone—their husbands and children remaining in India with the in-laws—and nothing can recover the days, weeks, and years lost to them through their physical absence. Here then is the irony and the sameness: that in meeting the filial responsibilities to care for elders, the challenges of delivering everyday physical care to someone else's parents are traded for the loneliness of virtual care to one's own parents. In reading this thoughtful and provocative book, we are left with troubled questions of the balance of the material and personal costs of care.

CALLING FAMILY

PART 1 MAPPING LANDSCAPES

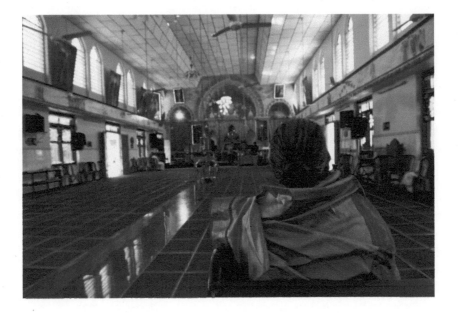

1 · ENACTING CARE

Health and care are often understood as two distinctive phenomena, with formal health care being separated from informal care along the lines of professionalization of skills and knowledge, financing, and public and private spheres of life. However, considering that ill health, infection, disease, and aging are social experiences, questions of health are inevitably questions of care. It is impossible to write about aging and its specific consequences for health without asking who provides everyday care, such as nourishment, bathing, and emotional support, and who provides care that is more obviously related to health, such as taking someone to or from doctor's appointments, purchasing and monitoring medication, and so on. Around the world, most care is provided informally, and health providers in both public and private sectors are summoned when such care is no longer enough. In this book, I aim to blur the problematic distinction between formal health care and informal care through inquiring what happens when the presumed conditions for what is locally understood as good eldercare are disrupted by geographic distance among family members. By doing so, I illuminate how care is shaped by people as well as by material objects such as digital technologies and money, particularly in the form of remittances. I approach this issue through the case study of nurses from Kerala, South India, who migrate abroad for work while their aging parents remain in India. This group of people is specific in several aspects, including its predominantly Syrian Christian background. Additionally, the migrating children who provide informal care at a distance are nurses and thus professional health-care workers. As such, they are well suited for a study of the blurring of the boundary between daily and health-specific care. Based on experiences of these families, this book investigates how digital technologies help to enact care within what I call transnational care collectives.

Off the main road leading to Kottayam, a district capital in central Kerala, jackfruit, coconut, and rubber trees abound. Through the window of the car that was taking me to an interview, the South India that I was just beginning to discover was a far cry from the images propagated by popular movies such as *Slumdog Millionaire* (2008). The houses hidden below the lush tropical foliage were anything but humble: comfortably spread out, with plenty of undulating land around each of them, they raised their pointed rooftops two or even three stories high. In the evening sun, these villas, painted in shades of ruby, sapphire, and citrine, sparkled like jewels nested in the green satin of their surroundings. Precious as they were, many of them were guarded by tall, steel double gates.

"Who lives here? What do the people here do to be able to construct such mansions?" I voiced my thoughts, astounded, as our car turned onto an offshoot lane. The polluted air of city traffic had gradually been replaced by a different kind of heaviness; the air was hot, humid, and pollen filled.

"It's all nurse money," Teresa explained indifferently. "Every household here has at least one person working as a nurse abroad."

Teresa would know—she used to be one of them. She had worked as a nurse in Oman for four years and then started the application process for a work visa in the United Kingdom.[1] Her fate and fortune as a successful migrant nurse abruptly came to a halt when her husband passed away in a car accident. Following this sudden tragedy, she decided to remain in Kerala. To sustain herself as a widowed mother of three, she changed her profession and established a popular beauty parlor, specializing in bridal services.

But now Teresa was taking me to the family of her friend Sara, another nurse who was still working in Oman at that time. Eventually, after meandering through abundant, privately owned pineapple fields, we turned onto a broad red-brick driveway. A two-story villa stood in front of us. The façade was partly covered with tiles, and the entrance was shielded by a typical Keralite terrace, *poomukham*, with a distinctive shiny teak railing. Attached to the entrance was another sloping roof, under which a small car covered with a protective cloth was parked. A couple of older people emerged from the house. These were Sara's parents, who welcomed us while Sara was busy in the Gulf, across the Arabian Sea. In the shade of the verandah, they looked too tiny to fill their enormous home.

"Tell the driver to follow the eastbound highway," Sara said to me on the phone. "But *I* am the driver," I replied, laughing.

Sara fell silent for a few moments, as she absorbed the idea of a woman driving by herself through the Omani desert in a rented car of dubious quality (figure 1.1). After gathering her thoughts, she continued to guide me to where she lived, in Shalim, a town some 180 miles (300 kilometers) from Muscat in central Oman. It was mid-October 2014, ten months after I had first met her parents. I had made few social connections in Muscat and found it challenging to engage with Indian nurses there, but when I phoned Sara she was eager to meet me: "Yes, I know you!" she said. "My parents told me all about you. Come and stay with me for two, three days!"

I readily accepted her invitation and left Muscat a couple of days later. The highway climbed some steep mountains, then descended into flat sand fields. There I passed several *wadis*, dry valleys that host streams, overflowing with

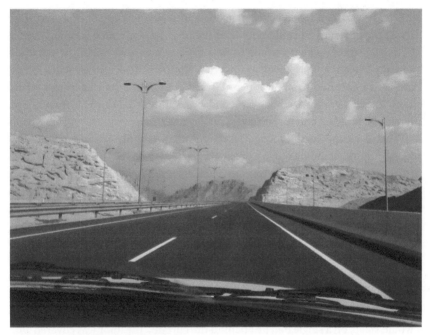

FIGURE 1.1. Driving through Oman.

violent torrents of water whenever it rains. I caught sight of my first camel, stripping tree leaves in front of a lonely house, partly hidden between two hills. The environment was moon-like—nothing but ochre gravel and rocks all around. The thermometer on my dashboard was a constant 122 degrees Fahrenheit (50 degrees Celsius), and I did not dare imagine what I would do if my car melted into a puddle on the road.

Shalim was a proper town, larger than I had expected to find in the middle of the barren land through which I traveled. The first white, flat-roofed buildings with tiny, sometimes arched windows slowly emerged from the sand ahead of me. In contrast to the gaudier styles of its Gulf neighbors, the architecture of Oman was minimalist and elegant, serving the needs of the residents populating the arid, sweltering environment. At a roundabout, sporting well-watered, carefully pruned greenery, I turned to the right onto the main road through Shalim. Skimming the surroundings in search of Sara's hospital, I noticed the many people walking on the pavements. They were mostly men, but many were not wearing *dishdasha*, the white long-sleeved garment that is the national Omani male dress. Instead, they wore brown, beige, and dark purple trousers and long shirts, known in much of South Asia as *kurta* or *panjabi*, implying that Shalim hosted a considerable number of migrants from that region.

I drove farther, past a row of shops, past a sign for a horse racing track and a market that was about to close; the sellers were rolling up their remaining rugs, and the buyers had loaded their newly acquired camels and sheep onto their Toyota pickup trucks. I could not locate the hospital, so I called Sara and parked at a supermarket in what seemed to be a town center. I waited in the car when suddenly I heard a loud knock against the window; a teenage boy with a shepherd's stick gestured to me to open it. I self-consciously refused—what could they make of a Western woman traveling alone at dusk? He and his friends simply smiled, nodded, and turned away.

When Sara appeared, I recognized her immediately. She was the only Indian woman around, standing out in a green *salwar kameez*, a typical Indian dress comprising of wide trousers and a tunic, with an essential *dupattā*, a shawl that covers the chest. Short and plump, she was strikingly like her mother. She hopped into the car and led me along a dusty side road. I parked and followed her through an ornately decorated heavy wooden door, into the secluded courtyard, and then into her apartment.

Sara lived here on her own, renting a spacious apartment on the ground floor of a house belonging to an important local family. The door opened into a large sitting area—"Seven people can sit here," Sara proudly noted—separated from the bedroom only by a thick curtain. Sara scurried behind it to show me where I would sleep, on a single bed just behind the curtain. The floor was covered with an old rug, but the ceiling seemed freshly painted and decorated with yellow and blue medallions and trim. A calendar hanging on an otherwise empty wall pictured a beautiful freshly painted house and a brand-new blue Hyundai. These were photographs of Sara's family house and car in Kerala. The calendar was a souvenir of the housewarming festivities for the investments that Sara's husband had made through her income; the loan for the renovation of his ancestral home would be repaid in the coming few years.

The bedroom windows were curtained, blocking any natural light. The room had no furniture other than two beds and a small table with a personal computer covered with a cloth. Noticing my quizzical look, Sara explained, "My uncle gave me this PC when he left Muscat. I used it for a while to talk to my family through the webcam, but now it's broken." She gestured *forget about it*—she had no intention of fixing the computer any time soon, and I wondered for a moment whether it was really broken. On the other hand, Sara happily exchanged photos, and loads of them, with her family in Kerala through WhatsApp on her smartphone.

As we sat on her couch, Sara took her phone and opened her Facebook application to show me photos of her "friends"—her co-workers at the hospital—but her family was nowhere to be seen. She explained that she did not post often at all on her Facebook wall. Rather, the photos posted there were by her friends who had tagged Sara to make sure she had seen them. But in her phone gallery, I could see plenty of photos downloaded from WhatsApp: there were a smiling friend who was a nurse in Europe, the newly renovated house in Kerala, and Sara at work, wearing her full nursing uniform and proudly posing in the operating theater. There were also plenty of photos of Sara's children, and a series of them from a shop where her daughter was trying on new salwari kurtas and asking Sara for advice on which dresses to buy.

I asked Sara whether these photos had the same emotional effect on her seeing her family live on the webcam, and she replied, cheerfully, "No, in the photos they are always smiling!" As we were sliding through the many snaps of Sara's children—at home, with their grandparents, at church events, in the school—I could observe that it was true: they always smiled. I realized that such was the very subtle impact of the photo lens, which was quite different from the webcam and therefore less emotionally demanding for a mother living far away all by herself.

From the sitting area, a wide hall, almost a room in itself, led to the kitchen. The hall was empty except for a tall refrigerator, a table, and a chair. Sara used the table to iron her clothes. To the right, there was a kitchenette with the sink so high that Sara had to stand on a wooden step stool to reach it comfortably. Next to the kitchen was a tiny, dilapidated bathroom. The electricity was not working well in there, but instead of trying to fix it, she had followed her husband's advice and bought a halogen light. Given that she lived alone, Sara said by way of explanation, it was wiser not to invite any men inside.

As the evening settled in, Sara told me about her daily life as a nurse in Shalim, where she had lived for over a decade. At 6:45 P.M. sharp, Sara checked the big clock hanging above the TV set: it was time to call her parents. She stood up to fetch her smartphone and then searched for Talkray, a free internet calling application that she had downloaded through the Google Play Store, because "everyone was talking about it." Her father picked up the call, and they talked for about ten minutes; he was most interested in how Sara was taking care of me and what we were going to have for dinner.

After Sara finished the call, she explained to me that she was always mindful of the time difference between the two countries—Kerala is 1.5 hours ahead of Oman. But she also considered the TV serials that her mother watched religiously and evening prayer times because her whole family were devout Syrian Christians. Sara called her parents, children, and husband daily, sometimes multiple times a day even if just for a few seconds. Among their conversation topics, health featured significantly.

"If there is anything related to illness, they will first discuss it with me," Sara said. "A while ago, the doctor in Kerala prescribed my mother some pills, and she started feeling dizzy after taking them. She first called me to ask about it, not her doctor. I looked for information about side effects on the internet, and I advised her to stop taking the pills. A week later she went to hospital, and she told the doctor, 'See, I stopped that medicine.' I told my mother, 'Don't tell him that I advised you to do so! If you do, he might get angry at my interfering with his treatment.' Sometimes doctors don't believe their patients when they report side effects. She told him everything, about the swelling, dizziness, constipation, all the side effects she had. She is allergic to some medicine, so I always take that into account. But the doctor told her, 'Only one in 100 people have such side effects, I can't believe it happened to you.' But my mother insisted, and he finally gave in, telling her to stop taking the pills."

Sara laughed. She was proud that she remained close to her parents across the many miles and years of living so far away, the evidence being her mother's trust in her advice.

What happens with eldercare when family members are separated through physical distance? This question is particularly pertinent in the contemporary world where physical separation between people is a fact of life for a number of reasons.[2] During the past few decades, people have been relocating nationally and internationally for work, studies, or love more frequently than ever before, stretching relationships across countries and continents. Among them, migrants from India have made their homeland a leading country of both out-migration and remittances.[3] In India and elsewhere, this trend has fueled a discourse of abandonment, which suggests that adult children neglect their aging parents in pursuit of a contemporary lifestyle that often necessitates mobility for work (Aboderin 2004; Shankardass and Rajan 2018; see chapter 3).

However, family members who are spread around the world often keep in touch through regular visiting as well as through digital technologies. In this way, families become transnational, separated from each other yet creating a "feeling of collective welfare and unity, i.e., 'familyhood,' even across national borders" (Bryceson and Vuorela 2002, 3). Considering the role of digital technologies in the making of transnational life, social science scholars have started challenging the idea that care without physical proximity is impossible (see, for example, Baldassar, Nedelcu, and Wilding 2016; Madianou and Miller 2012). Digital technologies, it has become clear, have turned out to be significant in sustaining family ties across geographic distance.

Then, in 2020, the COVID-19 pandemic hit. Consequently, all kinds of travel, including long-distance flights, were severely restrained and complicated through quarantine rules. Lockdowns and travel restrictions made regular visiting for transnational family members unfeasible. The measures adopted in many countries imposed physical distancing even among family members who lived within the same countries, cities, and villages. Following advice from medical experts, many governments considered aging people the most vulnerable, so they strongly advised this part of the population to limit socialization even with their children and grandchildren. Around the world, care institutions and nursing homes prevented their residents from being with family members to protect their physical health, with little regard to the impact of such measures on their quality of life and mental health (Gardner, States, and Bagley 2020; Roy et al. 2020; Grover et al. 2020). Digital technologies suddenly became additionally prominent mediators in family relationships, as they transpired as a preferred—and sometimes the single—alternative for family members to communicate and thereby maintain their relations. In the worst possible scenario, the webcam on a smartphone or iPad could even be the only means to say the final goodbye.

In this book, I further scholarly discussions on care at a distance by arguing that family members integrate digital technologies into their care practices, thereby forming global assemblages of human and nonhuman entities which I call transnational care collectives. This notion is grounded in the proposition that technologies such as mobile phones, smartphones, and social media are much more than tools that passively channel communication. Rather, digital devices and online platforms participate in transnational care collectives as active members, shaping what care comes to mean and how it should be done to be considered good. Given the increasing proliferation of digital technologies into every sphere of our lives, a trend which was additionally reinforced by the COVID-19 pandemic, there has never been a more vital moment to interrogate the subtle impact of technologies on people's lives, relationships, and identities. Care, a highly complex phenomenon that is essential to what it means to be human (Tronto 1993), is a prime domain for investigating the ways in which technologies influence how people relate to each other and who they come to be through their technologically mediated relationalities.

To a certain degree, social scientists have studied innovative technologies in the context of formal care, such as telemedicine and e-health.[4] But what of different types of everyday digital technologies such as phones and webcams? These devices are generic, readily available, and relatively accessible even to consumers from lower economic backgrounds. All over the world, digital technologies have become intimately integrated into people's lives (Miller et al. 2016) and, as I show in this book, into their everyday care practices. How do these technologies, then, influence how people understand care? How do they affect the ways in which people relate to each other through care, and even who they become? In this book, I address these questions by drawing on my ethnographic fieldwork, which I conducted intermittently between 2011 and 2022 with most intensive research periods in India and Oman in 2014 and 2015. I investigate my empirical data through material semiotics, a science and technology studies (STS) theoretical approach that I explain in greater detail later in this chapter.

TELEMEDICINE PILOTITIS

My interest in studying technologies in relation to care was sparked well before I ever set foot in India by an event that occurred in my home country, Slovenia. Between 2008 and 2009, I participated as a representative of a local health-care organization at several professional meetings on the topic of telemedicine development and implementation. The meetings were organized by the director of a major hospital who had assembled collaborators from private and public health-care sectors, academia, and the telecommunication industry to propose a plan for a national telemedicine program.

Sitting at a large round wooden table in an elegant conference room with about twenty people, I was struck by the discussion that took place that spring day. The focus of the conversation was mainly on how to strategically and convincingly present innovative technologies to the Minister of Health to secure funding. At no point was mention made of the people who would be required to use the proposed technological system—both health-care professionals and patients—or their specific needs.

As I became increasingly engaged with the field of telemedicine and e-health, I found that this sort of top-down approach was more of a rule than an exception. I joined several Med-e-Tel conferences, organized yearly in Luxembourg by the International Society for Telemedicine and eHealth (ISfTeH). Time and again I heard the presenters describe their highly innovative technological devices and systems as working "brilliantly" in the pilot stage. Difficulties inevitably occurred during the implementation at a larger scale, and the culprits for this were often claimed to be health-care professionals who reportedly refused to use the new technologies and stubbornly insisted on seeing their patients face to face.

During a coffee break, a leading member of ISfTeH, a slim, middle-aged man with a perfect tan, wearing a sleek gray suit, told me only half-jokingly that telemedicine was "suffering from chronic pilotitis"—that is, it was constantly stuck in the pilot phase, unable to become widely adopted at national and international levels. The reasons, according to him, were complex, including difficulties of interoperability, the inertia of governments to take telemedicine seriously, and the "culture" of health-care professionals that regarded physical co-presence as key to a proper medical examination. As I later strolled from one conference room to another, I could not help but wonder if the top-down approach, whereby a technological system is developed first then subsequently imposed on the people who are supposed to use it, was not a significant factor in persistent failures of telemedicine.

My hunch was confirmed when I discovered Jeannette Pols's book *Care at a Distance: On the Closeness of Technology* (2012), an ethnographic study of telemedicine implementation in the Netherlands. She clearly showed that telemonitoring—the use of technologies to follow chronic patients at a distance—did not exactly deliver on the promises of efficiency and reduced costs as the government had hoped. Rather, the telemonitoring system changed the nurses' routines and the required skills and knowledges: instead of traveling to their patients to check on them, nurses had to learn how take care of the technologies and how to deal with the data these devices produced.

The research I present in this book, and its focus on everyday digital technologies, is a reaction to what I was learning about telemedicine at that time. Instead of concentrating all efforts on technological innovation—which is often extremely expensive and demonstrably challenging to implement—what about looking at how care could be improved with commonplace, widely available and popular technologies? Instead of convincing people to adopt new technologies, why not learn from them how they are already using the devices they have at their fingertips for the purposes of care? How could the answers to these questions serve the people—both patients and health-care professionals—who at some point might need to rely on more sophisticated technologies for care?

BUILDING DISCIPLINARY BRIDGES

Theoretically, this book is a "generative interface" between anthropology and science and technology studies, or STS (Cadena et al. 2015). Such interfaces are sites where the practices, topics, and analytical tools of various disciplines come into conversation; they are generative in that they provide opportunities for establishing new, open-ended connections between different empirical and theoretical methodologies. Bringing together the research techniques of anthropology and STS care studies is a form of "bridgework," the intellectual work that scholars do to create possibilities for generative interfaces (Rodríguez-Muñiz 2016). Through bridgework, this book leads to novel understandings of what family care becomes when it is practiced in a transnational context with the help of digital technologies.

To start with, I build on earlier anthropological studies of migration, media, and communication that have explored digital technologies in transnational family care. Globally, the increased availability of information and communication devices has resulted in a significant decrease in the prices for telecommunication services, in better infrastructures, and in policies aimed at improving access to these technologies (Kilkey and Merla 2014). Readily accessible mobile phones have had a tremendous and multifaceted impact on families within India and those spanning the globe (Jeffrey and Doron 2013; Vertovec 2004).

In an effort to challenge the ideal of proximity in care, which rests on the assumption that geographic distance prohibits caregiving, Loretta Baldassar and her colleagues (2016) have argued that digital technologies indeed make care possible across space. Inspired by new materialism, particularly Jane Bennett's (2004) idea of "vibrant matter" which acknowledges the agency of materiality, this body of research has described how digital technologies enable transnational family members to produce various types of "co-presence," or the feeling of being together at a distance (Baldassar, Nedelcu, and Wilding 2016). Among them is "ordinary co-presence" with a further subtype of "ritual co-presence," which is established through brief, regular contact through digital technologies between transnational family members (Nedelcu and Wyss 2016). Ritual co-presence serves primarily to express basic solidarity through which migrating children accomplish their filial obligations. Another kind of ordinary co-presence is "omnipresent co-presence," or the sense of being together that is enabled through online digital technologies that combine audio and visual forms of communication and may be turned on continuously. Because video technologies afford the possibility to see another person, Mihaela Nedelcu and Malika Wyss (2016) suggest that this kind of co-presence is the closest to face-to-face interaction.

Co-presence is made possible and is variously shaped by "conditions of polymedia" (Baldassar 2016, 147), the combined uses of various kinds of digital technologies, through which families support communication and manage emotions. The notion of polymedia was initially proposed by Mirca Madianou and Daniel Miller (2012), who explored digital technology–mediated childcare provided by Filipina nurses living in the United Kingdom. In their study, people constantly switched among media that catered to different emotional registers: written messages and emails helped avoid confrontation, while children could experience frequent phone conversations as a form of distant surveillance by their mothers living abroad. Additionally, Madianou and Miller (2012) developed a theory of mediation that suggests digital technologies may highlight the tensions in family relationships that had existed prior to migration, and they may also help to preserve an "ideal distance" between parents and children that enhances their relationship. Specifically in relation to aging migrants, Loretta Baldassar and Raelene Wilding (2020) presented the concept of "digital kinning" to describe the process of engaging with new technologies to maintain familial support and social and cultural identities across geographic distance, with beneficial impact on the well-being of older migrants.

The literature I have briefly outlined shows that within the context of transnational family life, increasingly available, affordable, and accessible digital technologies have become key to care at a distance. This book contributes to the field by introducing the notion of transnational care collectives, which explores the specificities of how digital technologies participate in such care. In my analysis I draw on the material semiotic tools of STS care studies, according to which (1) care is something that humans and nonhumans enact through the relations they form with each other within practices aimed at improving a certain situation or at least keeping it stable; and (2) what is considered good care is a matter of practical accomplishments and tinkering rather than external ideals that people follow. I explain this in further detail in the next section.

ENACTING CARE THROUGH HETEROGENOUS RELATIONS

Imagine a person with flu-like symptoms, lying in a bed at home, not even able to get to her feet. A relative, or a friend, or a kindly neighbor comes in occasionally, carrying a cup of hot tea and some paracetamol. The only piece of medical equipment in the room is a thermometer, resting on the night table. Within a few days, her breathing becomes increasingly difficult. The postal service delivers an oximeter someone has ordered online, a tiny gadget that wraps around one's finger to measure blood oxygen saturation. Eventually someone decides it is time to call a doctor, and the doctor summons an ambulance.

At the hospital, the person transforms into a patient, who is moved immediately into an intensive care unit (ICU). The bed in this unit is nothing like the one at home; this one is equipped with countless buttons, power plugs, and cables that are connected to a bedside cardiac monitor, which records the patient's heart rate and rhythm, and to a blood pressure measuring device and other medical appliances. Equipped with complex technology, an ICU bed requires a specialized health-care staff to operate the machines which produce abstract images and sometimes alarming sounds. Not all health-care professionals have the knowledge to manage such a bed; even in hospitals where the number of ICU beds is sufficient, new patients may not be received because of the lack of staff who have the appropriate knowledge and skills to operate the beds (Karagiannidis et al. 2019; Summers 2020).

Care scholarship often treats people as exclusive agents in care, as caregivers or care-receivers (e.g., Tronto 1993). But care is radically different when enacted on a regular bed at home or on an ICU bed: these different types of beds involve distinctive technologies that in turn demand specific kinds of knowledges and skills of those around them. Thus, material objects shape care in significant ways, to the point where their involvement may become a question of life and death.

Compared with specialized health-care equipment, the influences of digital technologies on care are more challenging to uncover. After my first couple of months in Kerala, I attended an academic event with a number of anthropologists where I shared my fascination over how family members in my study called each other, only to hear one of my senior colleagues respond, "So people pick up the phone and call each other. What is so special about that?" Digital technologies have become so deeply engrained into many people's everyday life that we barely notice them. I argue that this concealed yet ubiquitous presence of digital technologies is precisely why it is important to start paying closer attention to them. To articulate a reply to my colleague's question, I have found STS helpful because this field offers the vocabulary and analytical tools which I could not locate within the anthropology of that time.

In STS care studies, care is analyzed as that which is enacted within specific practices (Mol 2002; Mol, Moser, and Pols 2010; Pols 2005). What makes care as enactment so interesting and different from other understandings of care, often drawn upon in studies of transnational care? Most of all, the notion of enactment proposes that objects are not stable entities that form relations with each other; rather, the very identity of every object is contingent on these relations. Following this line of thinking, the identity of objects is multiple: it shifts with every situation, with every new practice within which particular relations are formed (Mol 2002). Practices, then, are generative endeavors; they are "world-ing practices" as they continuously make the world and all its objects what they are (Blaser and de la Cadena 2018). The idea that what objects are or come to be—their ontology—is enacted through practices is therefore rather different from perspectivism whereby objects have an essential identity that people may observe from different perspectives.[5] This explains why interdisciplinarity is more challenging than often expected: such work is not only about adding together different perspectives on a particular object—for example, a certain medical condition—but also about understanding that the object in question is ontologically different in each discipline (Mol and Hardon 2020).

For example, in her book *The Body Multiple* (2002), Annemarie Mol shows how a disease like atherosclerosis becomes something else when it is enacted in the outpatient clinic, the laboratory, the pathology department, and other sites. In the consulting room, it is enacted primarily through the conversation in which the patient complains of "pain when walking" and answers the doctor's questions about this problem. In the laboratory, atherosclerosis is not so much about talk-ing but about taking measurements. Laboratory technicians and the various measuring tools they use together enact the disease either as a "fall in blood pres-sure" or an "increase in blood velocity." In the pathology department, atheroscle-rosis becomes yet something else; with the help of a microscope, it is enacted as "thickened blood vessel walls." In this way, an object is enacted differently in dif-ferent sites by different actors, who form relations with each other within differ-ent practices.

Following material semiotics, the relations through which something is enacted are heterogeneous because they are established between humans, objects, machines, and animals as well as organizations, ideas, and geographi-cal arrangements (Callon and Law 1997; Law 2009). Such "radical relationality" (Pols 2014) implies that technologies, too, are involved in the making of identi-ties within care practices because the identities of the actors are "not a given, but an outcome of their relations" (Pols 2014, 176; see also Haraway 1991).

Approaching objects as having a flexible identity that is shaped through het-erogenous relations is also a key difference between material semiotics and new materialism (Abrahamsson et al. 2015). To give an example, in their study of telecare in Spain, Daniel López and Miquel Domènech (2008) showed how an alarm pendant, which older people living alone can wear and touch to call for help in an emergency, enacts the users' bodies in different ways. Wearing the alarm device constantly enacts the user as having a "body-at-risk" because it makes users aware that their body might fail them at any moment. By contrast, when the user wears the pendant only occasionally, the body is enacted as "vig-orous" because the user still considers it to be capable of everyday activities.[6] In this way, human and nonhuman actors, and what they enact together, are not stable entities but are all mutable, fluid, and mutually dependent.

The material semiotic approach is particularly fruitful in studying care at a distance because it makes it possible to examine in depth the specificities of involving digital technologies—and other nonhuman actors, namely money—in transnational care. Globally, the increased availability of digital technologies has resulted in a significant decrease in the price of telecommunication services, better infrastructures, and policies aimed at improving access to digital technologies (Kilkey and Merla 2014). Cheap phone calls have been described as "a kind of social glue connecting small-scale social formations across the globe" (Vertovec 2004, 220). But what precisely is this glue, and how does it work? Material semiotics allow for an analysis of how people and digital technologies engage in mutual relations within specific practices through which they enact certain kinds of co-presence. So what precisely do people do with digital technologies to achieve the kind of co-presence that they interpret as care, or that can be recognized as care since it is intended to improve or maintain the well-being of those concerned in one way or another? And how do digital technologies shape this caring co-presence?

Further, to analyze how care at a distance may be perceived as good, I draw on empirical ethics, a derivative of material semiotics that explores how people strive to achieve "the good" in everyday care practices (Willems and Pols 2010). In health care, empirical ethics emerged as a reaction to normative ethical principles, covered in theoretical approaches such as care ethics (Tronto 1993), which may prove to be challenging to follow in practice (Willems and Pols 2010). The central proposition of empirical ethics is that rather than finding out how a certain practice aligns with particular normative views of care, attention should be paid to how people achieve some form of the good in care through daily tinkering. Again, this tinkering occurs not only among people but involving material things such as food, information technology (IT) systems, and specialized health-care machines that help people breathe (Mol, Moser, and Pols 2010). What good care means, then, is not so much a matter of following some fixed norms or ideals but is situated in and shaped by particular sociomaterial interactions as well as, I would add, by underlying emotions and affective relations.

Such an understanding of normativity presumes that norms are not stable imperatives but can potentially change under changing circumstances (Winance 2007). In cases of chronic illness, for example, good care is primarily not about finding a cure; that is (or presently may be) an impossible goal (Mol 2008). Instead, good care involves making small adjustments to achieve a good enough life—and sometimes fail at it—in the context of a specific chronic illness and its chronicity (Manderson and Smith-Morris 2010). To find out what good care is, empirical ethicists compare and contrast various practices to "consider and weigh what is the best way of living, or the least bad, for whom, and why" (Pols 2013, 23). What is good, then, is continuously and locally enacted through tinkering within heterogeneous relations, with "local" referring to the specific situations in which practices occur rather than to geographic regions (Yates-Doerr 2017).

Following the empirical ethics approach, I explore good care in terms of everyday "practical accomplishments" (Winance 2007, 631) through which people engage with digital technologies to find the best possible ways of "doing family" from a distance (Morgan 2011). Corresponding to the STS emphasis on practices, the notion of doing family explores family life as a set of activities, which moves away from seeing family as something static or in terms of positions and statuses (Morgan 2011, 6). In transnational families, attempts to do family are mediated through digital technologies, which are thereby essential to shaping good care across geographic distance.

With its emphasis on sociomaterial relations, the empirical ethics approach makes it possible to investigate daily calling as a care practice, leading to new understandings of how care can be good even when it is done from a distance. Comparing the practice of frequent calling across different digital devices helps to understand what kind of activity this is and under what conditions family members see it as a core component of good care.

TRANSNATIONAL CARE COLLECTIVES

Scholars of India have since long described family relations as integral to shaping the identity of family members (Brijnath 2014; Gregory 2011; Mines 1994; Sax 2009). In the Indian transnational families that I write about, these relations are further mediated through digital technologies. Yet, as I mentioned earlier, these devices are not merely passive tools of communication. Rather, digital technologies shape family care within what I call transnational care collectives. I take inspiration for this notion from Myriam Winance's analysis of care as it occurs within "a collective of humans and non-humans" (2010, 95).

Drawing on STS to study disability, Winance (2010) has shown how material objects such as wheelchairs become intricately involved in the relationship between a person with disability and their carer by changing the relations of dependency between them. A new wheelchair must be adapted to make it comfortable for use not only by the person with disability but also, importantly, by the carer who pushes the chair most of the time. These adjustments are done through tinkering, a process through which people "meticulously explore, 'quibble,' test, touch, adapt, adjust, pay attention to details and change them, until a suitable arrangement (material, emotional, relational) has been reached" (Winance 2010, 111).

In Winance's case study, tinkering was about experimenting with changing settings of the wheelchair to see which arrangement worked best for the implicated people. Can the seat be adjusted so that the person sitting in it does not feel any instability? Does a certain position of the handles cause the carer back pain? Can the chin control be positioned in a way that allows the person with cerebral motor deficiency to maneuver the wheelchair independently, at least sometimes? Understanding care as attention paid to sensations and the possibilities of action that appear through the relationships within a collective implies that the object of care is not a single person but the collective itself, and this includes the wheelchair.

Even though the person with disability and the carer do not have the same abilities, the care relationship between them is no longer one in which an active caregiver assists a passive care receiver. Instead, through testing, tinkering with, and adjusting the wheelchair, everyone in the collective is both giving and receiving care and adapting to one another so that they can live together and make the most of their situation. Although care is specific for each member of the collective, understanding care as an outcome of a heterogenous collaboration makes the balance among the participants slightly more symmetrical and enabling, compared with the framework of caregiving and care receiving (Winance 2010).[7]

In my work, I extend the idea of care as enacted within heterogenous collectives to another realm—that of family care at a distance—and to different kind of technologies, namely generic digital technologies rather than highly specialized health care devices. The notion of transnational care collectives serves to explore care in transnational contexts through the STS conceptualization of care, understood not so much in terms of caregiving and care receiving, but in terms of shared work that includes people and material objects such as digital technologies. As a result, the subtle impacts of these devices on care and family relations come to light; otherwise, they could easily have been overlooked.

Through transnational care collectives it is, for example, possible to observe how people tinker with multiple types of technologies, telecommunication infrastructures, work schedules, time zones, and social obligations to establish a dynamic that works for all members involved, human and nonhuman alike. It is possible to see how transnational care is enacted in the collective and how the collective is taken care of. Further, one can discern how various types of technologies such as phones and webcams lead to different ways in which people relate to one another in caring relations—or how a seemingly simple practice of frequent calling contributes to shifts in filial obligations, especially for daughters. The change from writing letters to calling home is thus more than just a shift in modes of communication. It brings about more fundamental changes to people's relationships as it influences how people see and position themselves and each other within their social structures—or, in other words, who they are. The small, everyday acts of picking up a phone or swiping a smartphone screen with a finger become involved in a radical reshaping of personal and communal identity. To uncover such impacts of digital technologies on individuals, and through them on communities at large, is the contribution of transnational care collectives.

Like care in transnational collectives, bridges work in more complex ways than unilateral directions, so it is not only the anthropological approach to transnational care that is enriched by STS theoretical approaches in this book. While the material semiotic analysis focuses on the role of materiality—of medical technologies and bodily sensations, for example—in enacting care, I found that transnational care collectives are significantly motivated by affect, specifically by affective relations between parents and their children, but also grandchildren, other family members, and, significantly, friends and neighbors. In my fieldwork, affect—that "primal energy flowing between people and attaching us to each other, our institutions, and our relationships . . . underpinning people's emotions, behaviors and actions" (McKay 2016, 5)—transpired as the fuel that led family members to establish transnational care collectives and the glue that kept them going.

Additionally, while attempting to avoid "geographical exceptionalism" (Raghuram 2012, 170), whereby care is understood as different in different places because it is shaped through different "cultures" or moral values, I show how everyday care practices are situated within specific "geohistories" that shape the "structural conditions of caring" (Raghuram 2016, 512). Empirical ethics, combined with anthropological insights about the patriarchal kinship system, the Syrian Christian ethics of care, and the migration patterns of nurses from Kerala, clarify how "good care" in transnational care collectives is shaped by particular histories, tied to certain geographic locations.

CHAPTER OVERVIEW

The first part of this book maps out the theoretical, empirical, and contextual landscapes that are relevant to the understanding of transnational care collectives as they are created among transnational families of mostly Syrian Christian nurses. Chapter 1 presents the conceptual field of material semiotics and empirical ethics, and chapter 2 describes the field sites of Kerala and Oman, outlining the broader social, political, demographic, and technological background of migrating nurses and their families. Methodologically, I initially envisaged my fieldwork as multisited, but digital technologies made my field site more complex than that. Taking participant observation seriously—along with the idea of tinkering—I welcomed the mobile phone and webcam into my methodology. Conducting observation and interviews through these devices with nurses around the world led me to reconsider the field as a geographic location, and I explore this through the concept of field events.

Paying further attention to the context of eldercare in Kerala, chapter 3 outlines the public discourse of abandonment, which presumes that older adults who do not live together with one of their children are deserted, neglected, and subject to pity. The ideal of co-residence can be broken through older people living in institutions, such as old age shelters, homes, and geriatric hospitals, which are consequently commonly seen as miserable places. Along the same lines, in the case of migration the parents are portrayed as left behind by their presumably individualistic, materially oriented migrating children. Among other venues, this discourse is reinforced through images on social media. I show, however, that the lived experiences of older adults who do not live the ideal of co-residence are much more multifaceted.

The second part of the book is dedicated to exploring transnational care collectives that challenge the discourse of abandonment through international migration. Without doubt, some practices, such as cooking, feeding, bathing, cleaning, and living under the same roof are indeed made impossible through geographic distance. I argue, however, that within transnational care collectives eldercare does not simply cease but is transformed as people find new ways to do care at a distance. In chapter 4 I show how, with the inclusion of digital technologies, care becomes enacted within practices such as frequent calling. Transnational care collectives are created through tinkering with various digital devices and sociopolitical contexts of telecommunication, calling routines, and kin and non-kin members who become included at different points in time, for different purposes and with different levels of intensity. These aspects shape the specific dynamic of each collective. Further, transnational care collectives are stimulated and maintained by affect, which also stimulates daily care for the digital technologies themselves. I illuminate how care in transnational collectives is shared among all its members, human and nonhuman alike, and I investigate how different types of technologies enable people to relate to each other in different ways.

The next two chapters look at the intricacies of care in transnational care collectives, first through the changes of what it means to be a good child, and especially a good daughter, and then specifically in relation to health. In this way, care practices that often remain unseen, and therefore undervalued, come to light as significantly related to health outcomes. In chapter 5, I investigate the influence of international migration on the filial obligations among Syrian Christian female nurses. Exploring eldercare practices highlights complex changes in gender dynamics and kin relations in a transnational context. Because they are tied to international migration, digital technologies and money, in its different forms, co-shape new norms of filial care by transforming the expectations of children, especially daughters. As migrating laborers, female nurses may increase their bargaining power with their in-laws in relation to caring for their own parents, and this may further influence the position of men as husbands and sons-in-law.

In chapter 6 care is investigated in relation to health: how are chronic illness, accidents, serious physical and mental deterioration, or a global pandemic dealt with in transnational care collectives? I pay attention to how digital technologies support families when dealing with various health conditions, and how they also may fail. Within transnational care collectives various tensions may arise, such as frictions among siblings who are trying to arrange physical care for a parent in need. Further, a comparison of photographs and live images that are transmitted through smartphones, laptops, and tablets illuminates the affective dimensions of caring at a distance and the "unbearable feelings" that some of these devices may produce. The chapter then addresses the question of return migration: if migrating abroad is a decision that adults make also with the view of taking care of their aging parents, what should they do when the parents are nearing the end of their life?

Finally, in the conclusion of the book I review the key aspects of transnational care collectives and consider some lessons that this work offers to those working in the field of technologies for health.

2 · CRAFTING THE FIELD

> For me, as for most Malayalis, there is Kerala and there is India. The two
> are one, of course, but Kerala is so different from the rest of the country
> and so unique in its landscape, culture and history that a Malayali grows
> up having a mental distinction between Kerala and the rest of India
> —Abraham 2002, 96.

Abu Abraham (2002) opens his essay on the history of Kerala by noting its distinctiveness. He emphasizes that Malayalis, as the people of Kerala
refer to themselves, feel strongly connected with the rest of India, especially
through Hindu traditions. But the state is also distinctive, as repeatedly highlighted in popular and academic discourse in and on India. As Robin Jeffrey
(2016) points out, Kerala stands out in many ways demographically and
socioeconomically: among other social indicators that make Kerala a "success,"
it has high life expectancy, low infant mortality rates, and almost universal literacy, including among women, all a consequence of the particular cocktail of
communism, Christianity, commercial connections, and historical matriliny
(Jefferey 2004).

The smallest of Indian states in terms of population and area, formally established in 1956, Kerala is often represented as a "model" state, praised for its economic development and achievements in health, education, and women's rights
(Thomas 2014).[1] This narrative emerged in the 1970s when a United Nations
study found that Kerala scored remarkably high on social indicators despite its
low economic growth (Devika 2010). While recognizing the exceptionally
strong "desire for development" among Malayalis (Gallo 2017, 17), scholars have
also attributed these extraordinary social indicators to the local politics. The
communist government came to power in Kerala through free ballot in 1957 and
subsequently developed a "democratic style of functioning" (Thomas 2014, 259),
with the state supporting grassroot movements and involving its citizens in
development and social change. The ubiquitous praise for Kerala's social tri-
umphs adds to its enigmatic character and powers the pride of Malayalis when
asked about their homeland.

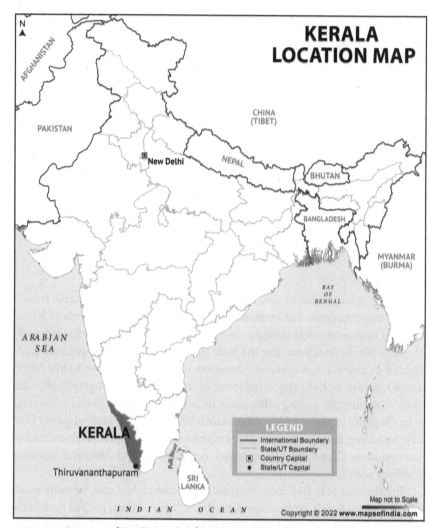

FIGURE 2.1. Location of Kerala in India. (Map reprinted courtesy of mapsofindia.com.)

Shaped like a tattered banana leaf, Kerala lies at the extreme southern tip of India (figures 2.1 and 2.2). To the east, it shares borders with the states of Tamil Nadu and Karnataka, separated by the Western Ghat, a cool and rugged mountain range that is older than the Himalayas. From there, the landscape unravels into rolling hills, which unfold into coastal lowlands. To the west, Kerala disappears into the Arabian Sea. In January 2014, before I landed in Kochi (also known as Cochin), a major port city in the southwest of the state, I had spent some time in Sri Lanka. I was struck by the similarity of the two places, at least at first sight. In both sites, temperatures rarely dropped below 70 degrees and often reached 100 degrees Fahrenheit (20 to almost 40 degrees Celsius), and the hot

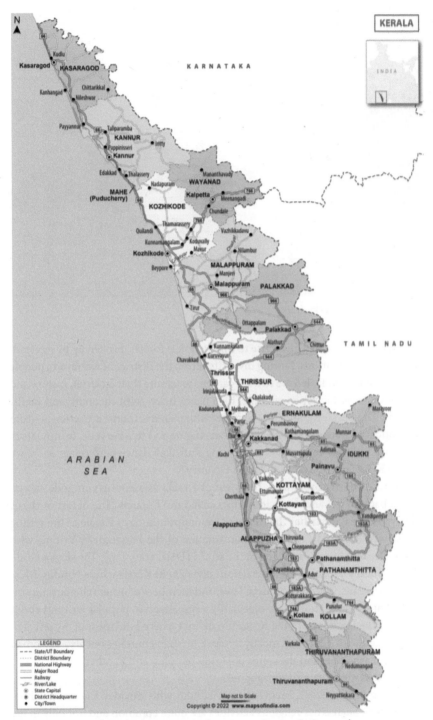

FIGURE 2.2. Map of Kerala. (Map reprinted courtesy of mapsofindia.com.)

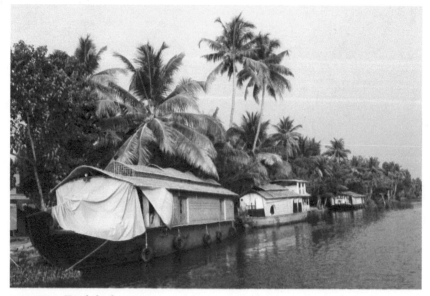

FIGURE 2.3. Kerala backwaters.

and humid climate had given rise to thick tropical forests, broken up by rice pad-
dies and tea plantations. During my visits across the district of Kottayam, people
regularly and proudly led me to their gardens to admire their jackfruit, cashew and
cinnamon trees, black pepper vines, high palms heavy with coconuts, and vanilla
orchids. This vegetal abundance, together with plentiful tourist attractions—from
romantic backwater cruises on houseboats (figure 2.3) to Ayurvedic treatments in
luxurious wellness centers and captivating Kathakali dance performances—have
earned Kerala the title of "God's Own Country."

Beyond tourist brochures, the view of Kerala as a country of gods can be
traced back to the ancient manuscripts called the Puranas. The oldest of these,
Matsya Purana, describes the Malaya Mountains in today's Kerala as the setting
of the meeting of Matsya, the first incarnation of the Hindu deity Vishnu, with
Manu, the first human and king of the world (Dalal 2010, 250). The slogan God's
Own Country evokes the wide religious diversity in Kerala where Hindus, Muslims, Christians, Sikhs, Buddhists, Jews, and members of other religious minorities cohabit—peacefully, as is repeatedly emphasized in popular writings about
Kerala.[2] The landscape of the Kottayam district where I did most of my research
was pierced with belfries of mostly Syrian Christian churches but also of Roman
Catholic cathedrals and the spires of Hindu temples, and in other districts I also
came across mosques and synagogues.

During my fieldwork, I regularly met Hindus who attended the Syrian Christian masses. Such cross-religious activities are quite common and not only in my
experience. In his essay on the history of Syrian Christianity in Kerala, William

Dalrymple (2002) describes an encounter with a Hindu woman who regularly prayed to St. Thomas. In 52 A.D., this apostle allegedly sailed from Palestine to Kerala where he started converting local Brahmins (members of the highest caste or *varna* in Hinduism) to Syrian Christianity, "a distinctively more Jewish form of the religion than that brought to Europe by St. Paul" at around the same time (Dalrymple 2002, 70).[3] Syrian Christians from Kerala, also called Saint Thomas Christians, claim descent from these first converts; the descriptor refers not to Syrian ancestry but to their Syrian liturgy (George 2005, 6). St. Thomas, whose existence and arrival to India remain disputed, was later opposed by orthodox Brahmins, and he was martyred at the ancient temple town of Mylapore in Tamil Nadu.

Although its congregation shares this origin story, Syrian Christianity in India has undergone multiple divisions, which over time have led to various factions, including Catholic, Orthodox, and Reformed, many with their own bishops. One of them, the Syro-Malabar Catholic Bishop of Kottayam, Mar Kuriakose Kunnacherry, reportedly said that "Kottayam is famous for coconuts and bishops" (Sprague 2002). Today, religious tolerance is hailed as one aspect that makes Kerala unique, not only in India but globally.[4]

PRESERVING PURITY

Syrian Christians, numbering about 6 million, are a demographic minority in India, and most of them reside in central Kerala. They have been described as privileged in terms of race, class, and caste; although the caste system is essentially embedded in Hinduism, it endures among Keralite Christians as well (Thomas 2018). Rather than stepping out of the caste system altogether, Syrian Christians have become integrated into it as a *jyati* or a subcaste (Viswanathan 1999, 2), with internal divisions grounded in a long history of splits and conversions under the influence of migrations from the Middle East and as a consequence of European colonial control.

The Syrian Orthodox Church in India is part of the Universal Syrian Orthodox Church, which emerged as an indigenous church in Syria and then spread around the world.[5] St. Thomas is believed to have baptized the first converts, originally Namboodiri Brahmins and matrilineal Nairs, members of the highest castes. This small Syrian Christian community settled in the northern part of Cranganore, a town on the Malabar coast. In 325 A.D., they were joined by about seventy Syrian Christian merchant families from Jerusalem and Syria who arrived under the guidance of Thomas de Cana (Thomas 2016, 105). These newcomers, known today as Knanaya, settled in southern Cranganore, and the two Syrian Christian groups came to be referred to as "the Northists" (*thekkan*) and "the Southists" (*vakakken*), respectively. Today, spatial separation of religious communities is no longer as marked, although closely knit neighborhoods affiliated with specific churches remain.

Both groups of these early Syrian Christians were traders and landowners who enjoyed the benevolence of Hindu kings due to their reputation for being hardworking and prosperous. In recognition of their good deeds and services to society, they were accorded the privileges and honors of a high caste (Viswanathan 1999), as reflected in titles such as *Pannikkar* (warrior), *Vaidyan* (doctor), and *Tharakkan* (tax collector). Contemporary Syrian Christian groups still claim membership in the upper caste of Indian society (Philips 2004).

In the sixteenth century, a major division among the Christians of Kerala occurred when Portuguese colonizers took over state reign. Portuguese Roman Catholic missionaries converted lower-class Hindus, mostly of the fisher castes, Mukkuvans and Arayas, to Christianity en masse. These newer Christians and the earlier Christians with whom they intermarried became known as Latin Catholics. Another major internal division occurred in the nineteenth and twentieth centuries under British colonial rule when European missionaries converted people from the lowest Hindu castes, the Dalits; they readily embraced Christianity in hopes of escaping the oppressive caste system.[6] This group became known as New Christians or Protestant Christians.

These divisions resulted in three major groupings, which Fuller (1976, 55) has suggested may be "sensibly regarded as castes." They are maintained through endogamous marriage rules which are especially strict among Knanaya; not following them, intentionally or not, may result in severe punishment and excommunication (Swiderski 1988; Reddy 2018; Phillips 2004). Intracaste and intrareligious marriages do occur but are fraught with sociopolitical tensions and are often considered as "fake" or "fictive" kinship (Gallo 2021). While deeming intracommunity marriage important, the church in general is usually not actively involved in helping families find marriage partners for their children. Instead, in recent years, marriage websites such as m4marry.com have become increasingly popular; among forty categories in the website search is the option "caste/denomination."

Caste has far from disappeared among Syrian Christians, and caste distinctions, tensions and discrimination remain a significant social issue (Ameerudheen 2018; see also Swiderski 1988). As Amali Philips (2004, 257) noted, endogamy is not a sufficient criterion to define caste; other important markers include genealogy, place of origin, time of conversion to Christianity, food habits, degree of communal solidarity, differences in dowry, occupation, education, and even mental health status. Occupation and education are intrinsically related to class. Upper-caste Syrian Christians, who trace their descent to Brahmins, Nairs (or Nayar), or the "pure" Syrian Christians, are generally the wealthiest, and Latin Catholics and New Christians who are associated with their Dalit origins tend to belong to the lower and middle classes (Fuller 1976; Viswanathan 1999).

Caste and class are important because they strongly influence the professions that people in India may practice. According to Hindu ideology, practices—and professions—that involve touching and dealing with bodily fluids are considered dirty and dangerous because they offer an opportunity for members of higher castes to become polluted by those of lower castes. Bearing this in mind, it is no coincidence that Dalits are also referred to as "untouchables" (Ray and Qayum 2009; Sax 2009). The management of physical contact is at the same time intimate and political because it supports the hierarchies of caste and of society in general (Goody [1982] 1996, 114–115).

Within this caste system, the nursing profession, which is at the center of this book, is doubly stigmatized: first, it involves close physical contact with non-kin patients of all castes, including during night shifts, and second, it is mostly practiced by women. Through their sexuality, women are considered both powerful and perilous; their contact with other people is risky and therefore deserves special attention. Adult men are especially vulnerable to contamination via women, leading to everyone in their caste losing status, property, and power (Sax 1991). For these reasons, nursing is not particularly respected among Hindus and is generally devalued as a profession in India. Its reputation has only recently marginally improved with the increasing bureaucratization of the profession (Ray 2019).

Despite strict endogamic marriage rules among some denominations, Christians are usually not concerned about caste pollution to the same degree as Hindus. Scholars studying the early Syrian Christians have even noted that this ethnic group acted as "pollution neutralizers," meaning that the objects they touched became purified and appropriate to use by members of higher castes (Viswanathan 1999; Philips 2004). This could be one reason why Christians in Kerala are relatively open to nursing. Significantly, the majority of nurses in India originate from Kerala, and religion plays a substantial role in this phenomenon. According to Elisabeth Simon (2009, 88), Christians comprise only 3 percent of the Indian population, yet they are 30 percent of Indian nurses.[7]

In India, women started enlisting as nurses after 1914 when British colonial forces, English missionaries, and mission hospitals actively and aggressively recruited them, promoting the image of nursing as a noble Christian service that adheres to the Christian values of piety, service, and femininity (George 2005, 41; Percot and Rajan 2007). This discourse of nursing as a humanitarian and honorable mission has long provided the basis for despicably low salaries: nursing was seen as a service that could only be paid through charity and donations rather than through proper wages (Biju 2013).

This also means that nursing has a rather ambiguous reputation. One very pious older Syrian Christian woman, for example, told me that she was passionate about becoming a nurse because she thought about it as service to other people and therefore to God. But her father disapproved, insisting that this profession was only "for poor families" who had "too many daughters." Such families would often send the eldest of their daughters to become a nurse to ease their burden of having to provide dowry for her at marriage (see chapter 5). Within the Christian community, nursing might not have been stigmatized in terms of caste, but it was nonetheless stigmatized as an occupation of lower classes.

THE L'S OF KOTTAYAM

On the second day of my fieldwork, I found myself sitting on the passenger seat of a small black Hyundai. I was being taken to the Kottayam police station. Neela, a young local professional, was taking me there in person to check if I had to formally register for the duration of my stay. Driving along the bustling city streets, eyes firmly on the road and her foot constantly on the brake, Neela said, laughing, "You have to know this: Kottayam is known for 3 L's—literacy, latex, and liquor." She went on to add, in a more serious tone, "Despite the good position that women have in this society, men would still yell at them when they see them drive."

Released from the police, where nobody seemed to be interested in my where-abouts or my reasons for staying in Kottayam, I went online and visited the official website of the city. It offered a list of L's that was a bit different from Neela's: liquor was prudently replaced by "legends and lakes," but latex remained. Kottayam, a district capital of over 350,000 people, is famous for its rubber trees; here, the Rubber Board has its main office and still oversees the latex industry in India.

Literacy, too, was noted, and for good reason. In Kerala, 96 percent of the population is literate, with the smallest national gap of 2 percent between the male and female levels of literacy (Manoj 2020).[8] Kottayam is lauded as the first town in India to achieve "100% literacy" as early as 1989, based on people knowing how to read and write their own name and address (*UCA News* Staff 1989). It is also the home of the first printing press, established in 1821. In this city, the first Malayalam-English and English-Malayalam dictionary was printed, and "the first and only" association of writers, authors, and publishers—Sahithya Pravar-thaka Co-operative Society (SPCS)—was founded (Government of Kerala 2021). Kerala vibrates with literary festivals, and Kottayam has its share. At one point, I was even honored as a guest speaker at one such event, standing on the podium next to Urvashi Butalia, a feminist writer, publisher, and activist flown in from Delhi for the occasion.

High literacy levels among women indicate their exceptional position in Kerala compared with other Indian states. Women may appear in public, speak to men, and show initiative, partly an outcome of a distinctive local history of matriliny, which developed around the eleventh century C.E. and was practiced by the Nairs (Jeffrey 2004). This has been linked to the widespread "matrilineal ethos" still evident in contemporary Kerala (De Jong 2011, 17). A prominent example of an empowered woman emerging from this context is Mary Roy, a divorced Syrian Christian, a women's rights activist, and an educator who challenged the Travancore Christian Succession Act. Her legal battle to be treated equally in inheritance to her brother resulted in changes in the local legal system, and daughters are now officially entitled to equal inheritance shares. In practice, however, many women remain reluctant to claim their inheritance in order to maintain peaceful family relations (De Jong 2011). High literacy alone does not necessarily translate into a higher status, and patriarchy still holds strong, especially among Syrian Christians (Mukhopadhyay 2007; Thomas 2018).[9] Women's status in Kerala is succinctly captured in Neela's comment: women may drive, but men still yell at them.

Despite what tourist brochures may say, not only coconut milk and wild forest honey flow in God's Own Country. In her novel *The God of Small Things* (2002), the renowned writer Arundhati Roy, daughter of Mary Roy, writes of the repugnant smells of factory sewage and feces coming from a river that passed a five-star hotel:

> The view from the hotel was beautiful, but here too the water was thick and toxic. *No Swimming* signs had been put up in stylish calligraphy. They had built a tall wall to screen off the slum.... There wasn't much they could do about the smell ... they knew, those clever Hotel People, that smelliness, like other people's poverty, was merely a matter of getting used to. (220)

Roy's work was awarded the Booker Prize, a high-profile literary award given annually for the best novel written in English and published in the United Kingdom or Ireland. But in Kerala it was derided by many with whom I discussed it. They disapproved of the way the novel presented Kerala, unveiling its misogyny, caste-based social discrimination, and intercaste relationships. They disapproved of the author, too; they judged her harshly because of her family history, marked by divorces and court disputes (see also Philips 2003).

Recent studies, which examined the Kerala Model of Development more critically, found that social and economic development had circumvented the poorest populations and reinforced rather than challenged unequal power relations (Raman 2010). In her article in the Indian weekly magazine *Outlook*, Soma Wadhwa (2004) fiercely argues that the images of Kerala as a model state are nothing less than a "hoax," countered by high levels of suicide, alcoholism, unemployment, crime rates, and violence against women.[10] In an edited volume of essays, fiction and poetry on Kerala, Anita Nair, another internationally acclaimed Keralite author, noted clear discrepancies between the connotations of God's Own Country and what is found beneath the surface. Like Nair (2002, ix), I invite my readers "to read between lines and see beyond what is on display, to probe beyond the surface and tap into the seams of everyday," to revel in the beauty of Kerala as well as "to decipher, if not appreciate, the conundrum that Kerala is."

MIGRATING MALAYALIS AND FLYING ANGELS

The local legends of Parasurma and Mahabali accord the right to Kerala land, since antiquity, to Namboodiri Brahmin families.[11] Yet the land was never theirs to keep; for the last 2,000 years, Kerala experienced numerous invasions, contacts and exchanges through trade, politics, and religion. As Abu Abraham (2002, 97) writes, the earliest travelers from the West to the Kerala coast were Arabs, probably in search of spices. They were followed by the Greeks of Alexandria, the Romans, the Muslims from Egypt and Iran, and, in the thirteenth century, the Chinese. In 1498, Vasco da Gama opened the door to Portuguese who, after some conflict, took over and dominated trade and governed Kerala for about 150 years. Subsequently, Kerala was a colony of the Dutch, the French, the Danes, and finally the British. Britain governed the indigenous states of Travancore, Cochin (Kochi), and Malabar in northern Kerala from 1791 until India finally declared independence in 1947. Ethnographic accounts report lively maritime trade along the Kozikhode (Calicut) district coast also after independence, mainly with Arabs and the British (Osella and Osella 2006, 2007; Riedel 2018). In this way, constant foreign influences have shaped Kerala and its contemporary economy, politics, and people, producing a particular kind of local cosmopolitanism.

Not only did the world come to Kerala, but Keralites are well traveled, too. As I was told time and again, legend has it that when Neil Armstrong landed on the moon, he was greeted there by a Malayali running a teashop. India is a top country in the world in terms of out-migration, and despite fluctuations Kerala is among the top Indian states in this regard, receiving the most (19 percent) of all household remittances in 2016–2017 (International Labour Organization 2018; Reserve Bank of India 2018). Recently, the Kerala Migration Survey indicated that approximately 2.1 million Keralites live around the world, with almost 16 percent of them being women (Rajan and Zachariah 2019).[12]

Among the people I encountered, complex family histories of living and working abroad were far more common among Keralites than among families in North India. To offer but one example, a man in his 90s whom I met told me that he had been employed in the army as a young man, lived in Dubai for a while, and worked in Singapore for over a decade. All his children were born there before the family returned to Kerala when the youngest child was a toddler. One of my interlocutor's sons had worked in Oman for several years, and his daughter also had lived there for over thirty years with her family before returning to Kerala upon her husband's retirement.

Among Kerala's numerous foreign connections and exchanges, those with the Gulf countries seem to have been the longest and the most intense. This is partly due to the geographical proximity of the two locations: a flight from Kochi, Kerala, to Muscat, Oman, takes about three and a half hours, and traveling by sea takes less than a week. But there are also religious connections between Indian Muslims and the Muslims of the Middle East (Hansen 2001; Vora 2013). Migration from Kerala to the Middle East increased rapidly after the discovery of oil in the 1970s, which resulted in a dramatic increase of economic capital for the Gulf countries. By 2018, as many as 1.9 million Keralites, or almost 90 percent of all

Kerala migrants, had "gone to the Gulf," mostly to the United Arab Emirates, in search of employment (Rajan and Zachariah 2012). As with other Gulf states, Oman has thus historically been linked especially to Kerala through trade and labor migration, involving Keralites of different socioeconomic backgrounds.

In recent decades, nursing has become a profession of choice for aspiring international migrants, providing an efficient strategy to increase one's economic status (Nair 2012). International nurse migration dates from the 1950s when work opportunities appeared in the United States, and recruitment started with the support of the Indian government as well as the Syrian Christian church (George 2005). This trend was followed by large-scale recruitment by Middle Eastern countries between 1960s and 1990s (Percot 2006, 2014; Percot and Rajan 2007) and, at around the same time, also by Europe, especially Germany and Italy (Percot 2012; Gallo 2005; Kodoth and Jacob 2013). At the time of my fieldwork, Keralite nurses were migrating primarily to English-speaking countries such as Australia, New Zealand, and the United Kingdom.

The ebbs and flows of Keralite nurse migration have been significantly influenced by global politics. This was most palpable in the context of Brexit in the United Kingdom. In Britain, this event resulted in a dramatic drop of nurses originating from the European Economic Area (EEA) and, simultaneously, a sharp increase in the number of nurses from India (*Economist* Staff 2020). As I learned during my fieldwork, nurses take great advantage of social media to share information about the ever-changing migration regulations, employment opportunities, and work conditions around the world.

In 2014, I asked Jacob, a teacher of English, how many of his students were nurses. Leaning on the wall, looking in the distance while a breeze was drifting through the windowless classroom, he said, "Out of all students, 90 percent are nurses, the rest want to study abroad. Out of these 90 percent, 25 percent are male. These number had increased because they had realized that becoming a nurse is one way to go abroad and earn money. They are with their eye to the West."

Migration studies suggest that from 20 percent to over 50 percent of Indian nursing graduates intend to seek overseas opportunities (Thomas 2006; Walton-Roberts 2010; Zachariah and Rajan 2015). In one study, as many as 81 percent of nurses aged 20 to 29 planned to do so (Thomas 2006). Among labor migrants from Kerala, nurses, especially women with Syrian Christian background, are particularly well represented. I was not able to find precise numbers for Indian nurses abroad, but according to some rather dated estimates approximately 40,000 to 60,000 nurses from Kerala work in the Gulf countries (Percot 2006, 43).

The nurses' motivation to migrate has been strengthened by international socioeconomic inequalities that fuel global care chains, "a series of personal links between people across the globe based on the paid or unpaid work of caring" (Hochschild 2000, 131). The theory of global care chains highlights the globally structured disparities of class, race, ethnicity, and gender that encourage the movements of (non)professional carers from economically poorer countries in the global south and east to the wealthier countries in the north and west. As an origin country, Kerala fits this model well, especially because it has been trying to follow the Philippine model of "nurse production for export" by establishing agencies for market regulation and labor recruitment (Yeates 2009, 179–180).[13] As Nicola Yeates reports, this endeavor has been supported by the Indian corporate health-care training system, including hospitals, which has promoted nurse migration as a "trillion dollar business opportunity."

The prospects of migrating, earning significantly better salaries abroad, and sending remittances home have made nursing a desirable profession especially among lower- and middle-class families, across genders and religions. Migration may interfere with caste, class, and gender hierarchies as well as with kin relations in various ways.[14] In Kerala, nursing has proven to be such an effective strategy for moving upward socioeconomically that this profession has even started to attract men and Hindus (Johnson, Green, and Maben 2014; Walton-Roberts 2012). As Jacob explained to me, men became interested in nursing because of so-called industrial nursing. This branch of nursing increased in popularity after labor regulations were instituted that required health-care staff to be present in certain work environments, particularly at oil platforms. Workers in such environments are predominantly male, and women are not encouraged to take these positions for "safety reasons," an expression implicitly referring to the danger of sexual harassment.

"There's a boy who was an industrial nurse in Qatar for nine months," said Jacob as the lunch break in the school was coming to an end. "There were eight male nurses there but had nothing to do. They just had to be there and take care of small injuries or illnesses, nothing much. So he resigned and returned to Kerala. Now he has his own shop just down the road from here."

Jacob's comment implies that nurses could make decisions about where in the world to live and what to do relatively easily, almost frivolously. Yet as I describe in chapters 5 and 6, for the nurses I encountered, especially female, this was hardly the case. Rather, for most of them migration was a long and strenuous process that was rarely a matter of individual decision, but an outcome of complex circumstances and stark choices.

DIGITAL FIRST

In India, digital technologies are widely available, although they are differently accessible and affordable to people in rural and urban areas (Pandey 2020). Even in the most remote northern part of the country during my preliminary fieldwork in 2011, I had no problem buying a Wi-Fi Net Setter, a small device that enabled me to go online in the most remote village under the Indian Himalayas. Most people I met there owned a mobile phone, no matter their age or gender.

My host mother, in her late 60s, had a simple Nokia. She was illiterate, but pushing the green and red buttons was all she needed to know in order to communicate with her family members while she worked far out in the fields.

Over the past decade, cellular coverage across India has become close to 100 percent, and the internet, while not always speedy, has also become all-encompassing (McKetta 2019). The spread of digital technologies has influenced business, politics, and everyday life in India in complex ways although promises of increased democratization and reduced inequalities have not (yet) been entirely fulfilled (Jeffrey and Doron 2013).

In the meantime, the Keralite government has been working intensely to be "the first" in digital technologies, too. Among all Indian states, Kerala has the highest mobile phone penetration (about 90 percent) and internet penetration: 20 percent of households are connected through broadband, and another 15 percent of the population are connected through mobile phones (Mathews 2018). According to the official census, 9.5 percent of households in Kerala owned desktop computers in 2011 (Thomas 2013).

Next to building the infrastructure for digital technologies, Kerala officials also want their state to achieve the highest rate of digital literacy, most recently through the Kerala State Digital Mission, with its slogan "I am also digital." When the Government of India launched its national campaign Digital India in 2014, Kerala was already at the forefront of all Indian states in terms of digital technology use and initiatives (Joju and Manoj 2019). In Kochi, I visited a branch office of HelpAge India, a nongovernmental organization supporting senior people, and there I found several shiny black personal computers lined up for interested older people to learn how to use them. Years later, when I emailed the office in search of some information, their response was followed by a straightforward request: "Please train two elderly people unrelated to you in digital literacy." It is no coincidence that the cover image of this book comes from an article, published in the *Times of India*, reporting on a four-day digital literacy course that was offered by HelpAge India (Menon 2018). The organization has also published a very accessible manual (complete with images) on how to use smartphones, which has been produced specifically with older adults in mind.[15]

Another example of thriving digital technology initiatives is IT@School, a project that aims to enhance computer-aided learning in secondary schools and thereby reduce digital inequalities through free distribution of software and training for teachers and students. Within seven years since it started in 2002, it covered as many as 8,000 secondary schools (Thomas 2014). Even more impressive, after trade unions such as the Kerala State Teacher's Association protested the use of privately owned Microsoft software in public education, the IT@School initiative adopted a free and open source–based public sector software running through the local language, Malayalam. According to Pradip Thomas (2014, 263), the success of this and similar initiatives in Kerala was only possible because of the local "tradition of state-people partnerships" grounded in Kerala's specific political history of democratic communism.

Another reason for the wide adoption of IT@School was its integration with other public initiatives, such as the Kerala government project Kudumbashree, which aimed to empower women through microfinancing (Devika and Thampi 2007). This alliance translated into over 150 IT@School units being led by women, a significant achievement given that women, along with senior citizens, remain the most excluded population from digitalization elsewhere in India and around the world (Cabalquinto and Ahlin 2021; Dutta 2015; Thomas 2014). As a place with a quickly developing digital landscape and infrastructure, Kerala therefore offered itself as an excellent place to study digital technologies for care.

ANTHROPOLOGIST SHAPING THE FIELD

As I note in chapter 1, my interest in technologies for care at a distance was sparked by (stalled) developments in telemedicine globally. Another significant impetus that guided my research interests was much more personal, and this led to the inquiry about technologies within the fields of eldercare, family and migration. How to manage a relationship with one's aging family members when living abroad and how to take care of each other at a distance are questions that I have been dealing with personally since I first left my own home country more than a decade ago, first as an exchange student in France, then as a graduate student in Germany and the Netherlands. My analysis of care at a distance is thus inspired and informed by my own background as a transnational family member. I am familiar with hopping on a plane for an impromptu visit to a grandmother in the hospital or to attend an aunt's funeral. I hold memories of the unbearable feeling of helplessness upon hearing of my mother's serious health condition when international travel was impossible due to COVID-19 lockdown measures. I have also observed, with joy and awe, my toddler fully engrossed in play with her grandparents through the webcam. As I discussed such experiences with my interlocutors, I learned not only from but with them about care through digital technologies.

The complexity of family care in South Asia first caught my attention in 2010 during my first three-month-long ethnographic fieldwork in North India. As a student and intern at a health-oriented nongovernmental organization, I found myself in a tiny roadside village at the foothills of the Himalayas, counting and storing colorful pills that were then distributed to patients by Maya, a local pharmacist. Through our friendship, I learned about the intertwining of health with care, kinship, gender, caste, and religion, as it is situated within a broader political, social, and economic context of regional development (Ahlin 2012, 2018). I found that Maya's health condition—being excessively thin—was related to her ideas, shaped by the geohistories of her surroundings, of what she deserved as a daughter who should observe certain filial duties. During this fieldwork, I was also introduced to the practice of arranged marriage, the rules of intergenerational co-residence, and the role of money in shaping daughters' filial obligations in India.

To deepen my investigation of family care at a distance, I shifted my ethnographic focus from the northern to the southern extreme of India. The misty mountain slopes with dirt roads were substituted by luscious landscapes of wide, lazy rivers, and the Hindu temples were joined by numerous churches. Yet the principal ideas of living together, sharing food, and providing financially for aging people were strikingly similar across my two fieldwork locations. With scores of international migrants, especially nurses, Kerala represented a prime case study to explore transnational care. Among many other destination countries for nurses, I chose Oman as another field site. After obtaining the ethical approval for this study from the University of Amsterdam in November 2013, I spent in total eight months in India and three in Oman. In both countries, I traveled by taxis, rented cars, and buses from urban to semi-urban, and rural sites, ranging from Oman's capital city of Muscat to the middle-sized town of Kottayam in Kerala, to smaller villages and towns in both countries. I also interviewed nurses working in the United Arab Emirates, Saudi Arabia, the United States, the United Kingdom, Australia, New Zealand, Germany, and Guyana when they returned to visit their families in Kerala during their yearly leave from work.

I met most nurses in a popular English language school where many of them were preparing for the International English Language Testing System (IELTS), an examination that is often required to migrate to English-speaking countries. Through personal connections, I was introduced to Jacob, a teacher who warmly welcomed me into his class. Before I knew it, I was involved in the education process, and I gladly accepted my impromptu role as a volunteer teacher. While I was helping students improve their English skills, they shared with me their stories, worries, and views on migration, eldercare, and family relations, individually or in groups, squeezing on wobbly wooden benches. Some of them invited me to their homes to meet their parents. Additionally, I was introduced to several families by an Ayurvedic doctor based outside Kottayam and through other relationships I formed while in Kerala.[16] Then, using the method of following the people (Marcus 1995), I visited the daughters from families I had met in Kerala while they were in Oman. Such connections, however brief, were crucial to my fieldwork in the Gulf because without a local sponsor it was next to impossible for me to find interlocutors by simply walking into pharmacies, hospitals, and churches in Muscat.

A vital connection was also the friendship that I formed with Elisa, a middle-aged, married, Syrian Christian teacher whom I engaged as my research assistant. Thanks to her background in terms of age, marital status, profession, and religion, as well as her impeccable social manners and sensitivity, we were both well accepted in every home we visited together. Through lengthy conversations, I coached her to become attentive to nuances in the meanings and practices of care that I was interested in. Our discussions of the home visits and interviews that we jointly conducted became rich ethnographic events in themselves (Yates-Doerr 2019).

In Kerala, English and Malayalam are both official languages. Most discussions I had with my interlocutors were in English, some were even in German with nurses who (had) lived in Germany. Most older people, however, only spoke Malayalam. With them, Elisa's assistance in carrying out conversations and providing English transcriptions was invaluable. I also drew on their children's improvised translations and on my own basic knowledge of Malayalam to make intuitive assumptions about the events and conversations around me. It is possible that some nuances in personal relations eluded me, but not being able to focus on the words that the family members exchanged among themselves helped me direct my attention to the materialities of these events and to what people did rather than said.

FIELD EVENTS

One evening in February 2014, I was sitting at the kitchen table in a family house in Kerala enjoying a quiet moment after dinner with Mary, a young nurse whom I met in the English language school, and her parents. Mary had two older sisters who already worked as nurses in the United Kingdom. Around 11:00 P.M., a ringing sound came suddenly from Mary's room, the familiar tune indicating a Skype call. Mary stood up to bring her laptop to the dining table. It was *Achacha*, as the middle daughter's husband is generally referred to in Malayalam. As soon as he appeared on the webcam, Mary introduced me to him and told me excitedly I should "Talk to him!" And so I found myself having about half an hour of chat with Achacha; among other things, I learned about his views on and experiences of caring for parents and in-laws at a distance.

When designing my research, I had never planned to conduct interviews via digital technologies, but this was just the first out of many similar events later in which I engaged in remote data collection. My Skype conversation with Achacha seemed uneventful, comparable to many other Skype chats I had had in the past with my own family members, friends, and colleagues. And yet when the call was completed I felt something strange had happened that I needed to wrap my head around. I had left my home country and traveled to India to be in the field. But once I reached my field site, I found myself spending time with my interlocutors online while they were physically situated in other geographic parts of the world. Suddenly, the field site encompassed more than India and Oman, the physical locations I was visiting in person. Instead, digital technologies helped me reach

Keralite nurses who lived in numerous countries around the globe; I started conducting participant observation and interviews on the webcam and phone with nurses living in the United States, the United Kingdom, Canada, Germany, the Maldives, and Australia. And I began to wonder what kind of field this was and what the role of digital technologies was in shaping it.

Including digital technologies in the practice of fieldwork was a particular methodological challenge. It led me to take these technologies seriously as participants in my research and to reconsider how they were shaping the field. I propose the term *field events* to refer to situations of ethnographic importance that are co-created by ethnographers, their study participants, and digital technologies (Ahlin and Li 2019). As co-creators of field events, digital technologies mediate the relationship between ethnographers and their study participants and thereby shape data collection in specific ways (see also Nguyen et al. 2021).

Ethnographers must be aware of what digital technologies can offer, such as the possibility of reaching people who are constantly on the move or scattered around the globe. But I argue that researchers also need to be attentive to how using these technologies changes the data they gather. Fieldwork is an embodied practice (Okely 2007; Pink et al. 2015), so not traveling to the study participants' locations at all means that certain information and social relations may remain unknown and unavailable to the ethnographer. People may be less willing to share uncomfortable experiences through digital technologies (see chapter 6); some things that might be observed in person—such as crying while or after talking to a family member on the phone—might not be reported during a remote interview.

Much like care in a transnational context, doing fieldwork through digital technologies involves considerable tinkering to establish what such fieldwork actually is, how it impacts the researcher's field, and how it should be done to be considered good. In classic ethnographic research, fieldwork is evaluated based on the ethnographer trying to achieve total immersion in the field through living within a certain community and engaging with participants in their daily activities for at least a year (Carsten 2012). Although the prospects of total immersion are always questionable (Massey 2003), digitally co-created field events additionally complicate the standards of good fieldwork based on spatial and temporal boundaries. When doing research with mobile, technology-savvy people, a combination of visiting the study participants by physically traveling to them and co-creating digitally supported field events offers itself as an attractive option.

Establishing the standards of such mixed fieldwork is nothing less than a "practical accomplishment" (Winance 2007). The possibility of field events thus calls on ethnographers to seriously, and collectively, reconsider what good fieldwork through digital technologies may be.

3 · STRUGGLING WITH ABANDONMENT

Upon arriving in Kerala in January 2014, I was told on multiple occasions that conducting research on eldercare among the transnational families of nurses would be "impossible." The large-scale migration of nurses from Kerala, and out of India altogether, had apparently been making the situation for their aging parents "pitiable." Educated upper- and middle-class people talked about parents living alone in tragic terms. They spoke of older adults increasingly being abandoned to substandard care in old age shelters, homes, and hospitals or to live-in maids or visiting nurses who took care of them without the loving attention that a child might provide.

"This is what is happening today," one man lamented, reminiscing about the old times when at least one of the children, preferably the youngest son and his wife, would stay in the parents' house or the ancestral home. When I expressed my wish to meet some of these older people living alone, he retorted, "They will never speak to you!"—insinuating that parents would not want to disclose their profound grief over missing their children and their own shame over their children deserting them. He continued, "These parents, they go here and there, boasting about their children, saying, 'My son is in America, my daughter is in the U.K.,' but actually they feel lonely and sad. But of course, they will never say that out loud! They will never complain about their own children."

The parents admitting feelings of loneliness and isolation would signal weakness. It would be an admission that their children were "bad children" who had abandoned them; and, perhaps, it would suggest that they were "bad parents" who had raised their children to be oriented toward cash rather than care.

Yet shortly after this discussion, I was able to interview Alice, a 71-year-old widow who lived by herself. Together with the young priest who had helped to arrange the meeting and Niti, a young professional who had accompanied me to help with translation, we drove out of Kottayam one fine Sunday afternoon. Following the priest's instructions, Niti turned right off the main road to a bumpy country lane. We passed some elegant villas; the plates on their iron gates indicated that one belonged to a doctor and another one to a neurologist. Alice's house was halfway up the hill, surrounded by rubber plants and coconut palms. As soon as Niti parked in the driveway in front of the two-story house, which was freshly painted lavender, Alice emerged from the house.

Alice was a small, plump woman with dark grey hair, rounded silver glasses, and a blue cotton "nighty," a comfortable, long dress that women in India commonly wear when doing chores around their home. As she led us inside her home, her bare feet made almost no sound on the white and gray marble floor. She seated the three of us on the couch with plates of dates, sweets, and nuts in front of us, and she took a plastic chair and sat right next to the open door in a light breeze.

The visit did not start well. The priest insisted on guiding the conversation "to practice English," but then he refused to translate my questions ("It's not appropriate to ask a lady about her age or income") or took the liberty to provide the answers instead of Alice. Annoyed by this, I looked at Niti who sat next to me, quiet as a church mouse and visibly bored out of her mind. After a brief while, when Alice stood up to fetch watermelon juice from the kitchen, I nudged Niti and whispered to her that she, too, could speak. She took the cue and quickly followed Alice into the kitchen. When they returned, the two women were chatting merrily, as if they were old friends. The priest sunk further into the soft couch, but I did not care. Finally, I was hearing the stories I was after.

Alice had lived alone since her husband had died three years earlier from a heart attack. Her daughter, a nurse, lived with her own family in Australia, and her son and his family lived in Dubai. Not only did Alice say she was very satisfied with her life, but she also looked "genuinely happy," as Niti later described her. "I thought she would be sitting around, sulking all day!" Niti added, astonished.

The only time during our conversation that Alice revealed any sign of distress and loss was in relation to her deceased husband. Tears filled her eyes at the photos of him in the family album she was showing us. But when confronted directly with the question of how she felt about her living situation, Alice offered a very pragmatic explanation: "Because my children are abroad, I am living happily here. If they lived here and had no jobs or earned a very poor salary, would we all be happy? No!"

From Alice's answer it was clear that for her, just like in many other transnational families from the global south, "financial necessity trumped emotional concerns" (Gamburd 2008, 10). As my question was being translated for Alice, I could sense a sudden wave of irritation washing over her, and I wondered how often she had to defend herself and her children against insinuations of abandonment. Instead of being a victim, Alice attributed her positive emotional state to the practical benefits of having children abroad. Her children provided for her through remittances, which met her everyday living costs and had been used to renovate the house. Because she remained in the environment where she had lived for much of her life rather than following one of her children abroad, Alice had a lively social life. She attended mass at her local church regularly, and she was an active member of a women's association in her parish.

In the midst of our more than two hours of conversation, two men joined us in the sitting area briefly to personally invite Alice to the wedding of one of their relatives. She also found great joy in tending her garden, where she led us next. After admiring the rich variety of plants around her house, we stopped in the driveway where a small car was parked, protected with a car cover. Alice did not drive; the car was there for her children to use when they visited her yearly, each for a month. Besides their annual visits, they both called her on the phone every day. The obvious financial, social, and personal benefits for Alice were a worthwhile trade-off for not having her children living geographically nearby.

And thus I stumbled into the complex territory of diaspora and its management in relation to care for older adults in Kerala. The popular claims of abandonment through international migration were met with the lived experiences that suggested a more complicated picture. Although migration entailed leaving one's parents in a country with limited accessible formal infrastructure catering to older adults, and although the ideal of the cohabitation of parents and children persisted, many young adults left anyway. How was this situation managed?

Anthropologists have argued that kin relationships in India are strong because they are created through embodied activities such as daily eating and living together; these practices have even been described as co-constitutive of personhood (Lamb 1997; Mines 1994; Raval and Kral 2004). Among some communities in east-central India kin and non-kin are distinguished through tactile and non-tactile greetings, making physical touch a defining feature of kinship. For these communities, practices related to touching are so important that Chris Gregory (2011) has suggested the notion of "skinship" as an analytical category that brings together touch and kinship. Does such significance of physical touch for kinship mean that Indian transnational families at large disintegrate when they become extended across extensive geographic distances? If not, how do they manage physical separation among family members and maintain kinship ties?

To fully grasp how care is reshaped in a transnational context through digital technologies and money, as I argue throughout this book, it is first necessary to understand what is commonly thought to be good eldercare. In Kerala and more widely in India this is primarily achieved through intergenerational co-residence (Rajan and Kumar 2003). To illuminate the significance of this ideal of eldercare, Harold Garfinkel's ([1967] 1990) methodology of breaching experiment, which suggests that norms are best exposed when people deviate from them, is a fruitful approach. Generally, families may fail to co-reside in two cases, through institutionalized eldercare and intergenerational migration. In popular discourse, both situations are perceived as elder abandonment, and the families who engage in them are commonly labeled as "bad families" (Lamb 2000, 90).

In what follows, I first reveal layer upon layer of this discourse of elder abandonment by analyzing relevant images that I have found circulating on social media. Related discourses, such as those reinforcing the stigmatization of (especially female) labor migrants, may be found across the media, in films, and in literature and newspaper articles. To offer but one example, *Dollar* (1993), a Malayali movie directed by Raju Joseph that features a Keralite nurse working in the United States, conveys the message that money corrupts people and leads them to neglect their most important kinship obligations. My analysis, however, focuses on social media to show how digital technologies are implicated in shaping eldercare by reinforcing the ideal of intergenerational co-residence.

I then present the experience of parents who actually live in institutionalized eldercare and of those who co-reside with their children. Examining institutional care reveals how money as a hallmark of social class plays an important role in enacting residents of these institutions as either abandoned (if poor) or agentive (if well-to-do). By indicating how digital technologies and money are involved in eldercare, I paint the background against which the families of nurses conceptualize good eldercare in a transnational context.

THE CRISIS OF CARE

In English, one of two official languages in Kerala, one definition of the verb "to abandon," according to the *Oxford English Dictionary* (2021), is "to desert or forsake (a place, person, or cause); to leave behind; to leave without help or support."[1] Although the phrase "left behind" is not necessarily the equivalent of abandonment, it is often used in academic and policy discourses on transnational families in which young children and aging parents are presented as dependent on emigrant adults (Shankardass and Rajan 2018; Sørensen and Vammen 2014; United Nations 1999).

In the daily press in India, and in Kerala specifically, stories of the devastating fate of abandoned older people appear regularly. For instance, in July 2014 an English-language daily newspaper *The Hindu* published a story about three older sisters from Kerala who "had no one to take care of them" (Surendranath 2014). They lived alone on their government pensions until the eldest of them died. Her body lay at the house for two days before the neighbors found out and informed the police. The two remaining sisters were subsequently moved to a local Government Mental Health Centre. The article offered no details about these women's children or other relatives, but it used their example to present aging people living alone as being "abandoned" by their family members:

Increasing Number of Elderly Abandoned by Family: Situation Reflects the Break-down of Systems to Take Care of the Aged in Society

Increasing numbers of people are being abandoned by their families and forced to fend for themselves in their old age, social activists observed. "What happened to the sisters and other stories we hear about old people being abandoned at Guruvayur are all early warnings of a problem that is growing every day," said Biju Mathew, state head of HelpAge India. . . .

Social workers trying to bring relief to the elderly come across several cases where the elderly are left to fend for themselves as their children cannot take care of them. "In many cases, the children are working in different places or do not have the time or money to take care of the parents," said Nisha Varghese, co-ordinator of the Kerala Social Security Mission's Vayomithram project in Kochi. In such cases, Vayomithram helps shift the abandoned elderly to old-aged homes.

The story highlights the rapidly aging population in the context of insufficient state and family support for older people.[2] Across India, the proportion of older people is highest in Kerala, at around 12 percent of the state population, while mortality and fertility rates are by far the lowest of all Indian states (James et al. 2013; Philip 2011; Planning Commission of the Government of India 2008). The "breakdown of systems" of eldercare in the title of this news piece refers to the governmental system, which lacks provisions for health care, pensions, and old age home infrastructure, and to the conventional system of family eldercare, which is collapsing because of poverty and migration, internal and international. Neither system, government nor family, is deemed sufficient to cater to the increasing number of aging people in Kerala.

Others, too, have pointed to the fact that India lacks economic and social policies to manage the "exponential growth" of its aging population (e.g., Datta 2018). Years-long efforts have led to the introduction of various retirement and pension benefit schemes, but because of specific eligibility criteria these cover only about one-quarter of people in Kerala, with far fewer women than men receiving benefits (James et al. 2013).[3] Like in the case of health insurance plans, government-sponsored schemes target only selected portions of the population, such as those living below the poverty line (Ahlin, Nichter, and Pillai 2016; Narayana 2019). Often, the pensions are too low to allow for a tranquil retirement (Sampat and Dey 2017). This leaves those who live just above the poverty line in much financial distress, ineligible for state support and struggling to meet their living expenses. The increasing health expenses that usually accompany aging often add to their misfortune.[4]

Adult children, even if well-educated, may themselves experience financial problems, so their parents may be forced to work well into their old age or perhaps until their demise.[5] In case the children migrate for work—as is common in Kerala—they are often criticized for leaving their aging parents behind (Lamb

2009, 85; 2013). Many come to see them as "semi-absent" children who are either "materially present . . . [but] physically far away and unable to deliver love and care at close proximity, or physically nearby but materially unable to support their elderly family members" (Hromadžić 2018, 165). The idea underlying such "crisis of care" (Hromadzić 2018), which depicts aging people as neglected by their families and by the state, is that all care necessarily requires physical proximity.

MEMEFICATION OF CARE AND MIGRATION

Eating with Others, yet Alone

As the heat of the day gradually subsided and the dusk was falling across the Omani desert, I sat in Sara's living room, and I asked her what good care for parents meant for her and for people in Kerala generally. By way of replying, she unlocked her smartphone to share with me several memes that she came across through various social media channels. In one meme, which had reached her through a family group on WhatsApp, a group of older men were eating a meal in what appears to be a canteen. The men were all wearing white shirts, and they were eating with their hands from tin plates and drinking from tin cups. The words in the meme were translated to me as follows: "They are also parents of people like us! They worked hard to bring you up, to get you your preferred profession, even got you married to the spouse of your choice! And what did you give in return? Old age home! Remember, you will also have children one day!"

The central activity in this meme was eating, and this focus is significant. Across societies, food is rarely, if ever, just about providing physical nutrients to one's body. The way food is obtained, prepared, distributed, shared, and consumed represents "a system of communication" (Barthes 1975, 50), relative to specific contexts in which power relationships, gender, identity, and kinship are constituted through food-related practices (e.g., Manderson 1986; Carsten 1995). The importance of sharing food as a sign of charity and hospitality has been noted in historic Indian legal codes and epics as *danadharma* or the "law of the gift" whereby it is "the nature of food to be shared" (Mauss 1969, 73). People in India experience themselves to an important extent in the context of continuous exchanges of food with people and places that surround them (Ahlin 2018; Appadurai 1981; Barrett 2008; Marriott 1968; Sax 2009). Among Hindus in particular the exchange of food is at the same time intimate and political: the rules of food sharing are related to individual and group identity, and thereby to caste hierarchy (Goody [1982] 1996, 114–115).

As such, food is implicated in age, gender, and caste hierarchies as well as in what good eldercare means, and preparing and sharing food with one's parents has been described as "perhaps the most fundamental of all filial obligations" (Lamb 2000, 50). As Sarah Lamb explains, in childhood everyone incurs a moral debt through the food that their parents provide for them. This obliges children to participate in long-term or deferred reciprocity, whereby they are expected to provide nourishment for their parents in old age. Through cooking for their parents, adult children thus reciprocate for the physical and emotional nurturing they received in childhood. The cycle of reciprocity among family members is reflected in the meme Sara showed me, both through the visual reference to eating as well as in the caption.

Preparing food for others requires physical proximity, which makes co-residence with one's parents a critical filial obligation and a practical necessity. Across India, intergenerational co-residence is so essential to the ideal of good eldercare that it does not even need to be mentioned explicitly. The caption in the first meme that Sara shared with me implied that the image was taken at an old age home, and this was accentuated by the absence of children. Good children, the meme suggested, do not place their aging parents in an old age home; rather, their parents stay with one of them—or at least that is how it should be. In the case of several siblings, the preference is for the parents to stay with their oldest son in North India (Lamb 2000), although I was told that in Kerala the parents should stay with their youngest son.[6]

Two of the most essential and interrelated practices of good eldercare in Kerala, and across India, thus come to the fore: living together and preparing and sharing food. Through these practices, conviviality and nurturance as essential aspects of eldercare are sustained.

Only Near Is Dear

The idea that physical proximity is a crucial part of good eldercare is reinforced rather explicitly in memes shared through social media, such as another one that reached Sara through her Facebook page. Appealing to emotions by invoking nostalgic memories of childhood, this meme underlined the importance of intergenerational reciprocity as a moral duty. The necessity of physical proximity to fulfill that duty properly was highlighted in the caption referring to a parent holding a child's hands to teach them how to walk, and it was also evoked through the image of a younger hand holding and supporting an older hand. The words in the meme translate as follows: "I will not leave this hand simply . . . I learned to smile from my mother's face . . . With the help of my father's hands I learned to walk! They worked hard so that I live a comfortable life now! Because of all of this, the place of my parents is in my home (house/heart), not in an old age home or anywhere else!!!"

The word ഇടം (iṭaṁ) can be literally translated as "space," but several native speakers offered different possible interpretations. Most of them translated it as "home," and one suggested "heart/home." Like the notion of skinship, emphasizing the significance of touch for kinship among Halbi speakers in Chhattisgarh state in east-central India (Gregory 2011), this translation highlights the inseparability of physical and emotional closeness. Co-residence is care.

In a comment above the meme on Facebook, Sara had typed the words "Yes, of course," noting that she agreed with the message. An intriguing contradiction thus arises. Why would a nurse who left her parents in Kerala share an image that emphasizes the importance of physical proximity for good eldercare? Why would she reinforce the ideal of co-residence from which she herself had diverted? From my conversations with Sara and other nurses, it became clear that their decision to move abroad was not a matter of their individual choice but a long-planned family strategy, tied to what many perceived as poor living and work conditions at home (see chapter 5). Such distribution of agency among family members made the load of responsibility for taking the flight abroad lighter on nurses. Moreover, in India, and among migrant Indian women in particular, Facebook tends to be perceived as a place of public interaction (Gajjala and Verma 2018). By sharing the image on this platform, Sara was demonstrating to the public beyond her immediate family that she has not lost her moral compass on leaving her homeland.

The idea that geographic distance between family members automatically translates into the impossibility of all kinds of caregiving comes to the fore in the context of international migration. An article on LinkedIn, a social media website for professional networking, describes the "PICA (parents in India, children abroad) syndrome" as "a horrific emerging reality in urban India" (Krishnamoorthy 2015; see also Brijnath 2014, 7). According to the author, a medical doctor based in Tamil Nadu, South India, aging parents who are afflicted with this syndrome—and with serious physical conditions such as dementia—are left to live and die alone, and even their children's visits provide little comfort. In this gloomy picture, the children's migration is presented as a major cause of abandonment and is considered detrimental to the parents' well-being. At least some scholars agree, arguing that the out-migration of children from India, especially of adult sons, could be related to a higher risk of chronic disease for their parents due to the lack of physical support and the emotional distress over their children living away (Falkingham et al. 2017). Similarly, two images that Sara received through WhatsApp shape this discourse of elder abandonment in a transnational context.

The first image was a cartoon that features an older couple standing in the middle between their two migrating sons and their wives. The son standing to the left of his parents says to them, "I will take you, Mother, with us to Dubai"; his wife, standing next to him, is thinking to herself, "So we will have someone in the kitchen instead of a maid." The son standing to the right of his parents says, "Father, you will come with me to America"; his wife is thinking to herself, "So we will have someone to take care of our children while we are at work." After hearing their sons, the old couple decides otherwise: in the second part of the meme, they walk away with a scruffy bag in hand, following a sign which says, "Old Age Home Karunya Nilayam" (literally, "the house of kindness"). The father exclaims, "Old age home is better than our sons and their wives. If we go to there, at least we will be able to live together until we die!"

As I show later in this chapter, some older people in India do choose to live in old age institutions (see also Lamb 2000, 2009; Vatuk 1990). Yet the cartoon suggested that such a move by the parents is not completely voluntary but is precipitated by and in reaction to their "bad children." Like the movie *Dollar* (1993), the cartoon critically presents migrants as selfish, concerned only with their own needs, and far from the ideals of good children who take proper care of their parents. The implication here is that children who migrate do so primarily to increase their own economic capital, as reflected by the posh clothes and sunglasses worn by the sons in the cartoon. Furthermore, they invite their parents to live with them abroad not out of feelings of filial obligation, responsibility, and love but because they need a housekeeper and a babysitter. Arrogance, individualism, and materialism are thus embedded in the public discourses of international migrants.

This discourse applies to migrating nurses, too, as I found one Sunday afternoon in Kerala during a shopping spree with Jyoti, a middle-aged doctor I had met in the karate class in which I had enrolled (I joined for exercise, she for self-protection training). The sun was about to set when we entered an upmarket multilevel store that catered exclusively to women, and we lost our way among countless rows of colorful saris, bangles, and gold jewelry crammed across white, shiny tiles. While I was busy trying on *kurtis*, long, loose shirts that I actually knew how to wear (in contrast to saris), Jyoti was occupied with observing the other customers. As we were queuing at the payment counter, she made a barely visible gesture with her head to bring my attention to the woman in front of us.

"Look at her, what do you think her profession is?" Jyoti asked me, whispering.

"No idea," I whispered back.

"I bet she's a nurse working abroad," my friend mumbled.

"Oh? What makes you say that?"

"Just look at her, buying clothes so lavishly! And when picking them, she was ordering the shopkeepers around—give me two of these, two of those! So arrogant!"

I was surprised by Jyoti's observation and interpretation. In my eyes, the woman was just buying clothes like any other woman in the store, and she did not buy that many at all. She carried two shopping bags, none as full as mine. What was perfectly acceptable for me, a foreigner, was outrageous, from Jyoti's perspective, for a local woman who could be a nurse. The woman in the store perfectly fit Jyoti's stereotype of an arrogant, materialistic international labor migrant.

Memes that co-construct the negative discourse of international migrants and their families are also suggestive about their socioeconomic background. A final meme that Sara shared with me indicated that families who use migration as a strategy to improve their economic status are represented as essentially poor—and Christian. On the left, a visibly poor family with five children stands in front of a wooden shack; the parents pray, "Jesus! Please send at least one of these children to America, so that we can improve our lives." On the right, a change in the transnational family's economic standing is depicted: a luxurious new house, complete with a car, but the woman standing in front of the house is an old widow with no children around. She prays, "Oh Jesus! Please let at least one of the children return so we have somebody around to give us some hot water to drink!"

Memes like this one may be quite confronting for nurses from Kerala working abroad because they may easily recognize themselves in them. After all, they originate from families of the lower- or middle-class, and, as I have described in the chapter 2, they mostly come from Syrian Christian families. Because the history of nurse migration is so closely interrelated with a certain socioeconomic background as well as desired and realized upward class mobility, Syrian Christians are often described as more materialistic than the members of other religious communities. As one of my Hindu interlocutors commented, "On a Sunday, when you pass a church, what do you see? You see there are plenty of cars everywhere. When you go to a Hindu temple, you don't see any of that."

Yet Jyoti's comments in the department store indicate that the stereotyping occurs not only between different religious communities, but also within them. Not all Syrian Christians are necessarily regarded as materialistic, arrogant, and individualistic, but the nurses who migrate abroad for work may well be perceived as such. Among Syrian Christians, such labeling runs along the lines of class and migration status, which are both closely linked to profession. In contemporary hierarchies in Kerala, doctors, lawyers, and engineers are at the top, while nurses are in the middle or even lower parts of the professional echelon (see chapter 2). This hierarchy is generally reflected in local salaries and education fees for different degrees. However, migrating nurses disturb this order by having substantially higher salaries, not only compared to locally employed nurses but also to doctors, lawyers, and other high-level professionals. Jyoti was stunned to learn that a nurse in a Gulf country could earn 80,000 Indian rupees per month (about USD 1,100, according to conversion rates in 2021), while she herself made only about INR 60,000 (about USD 800) as a doctor. Reflecting on our conversation during shopping, I could not help but wonder whether Jyoti's resentment of migrant nurses stemmed least in part from the breach of local socioeconomic hierarchies that these nurses represented.

Images that are displayed in the press, on television, and through memes shared on social media "convey particular claims and define what are appropriate thoughts, actions and roles for members of society" (Xu 2020, 17; Gorham 1999). A visual cross-platform analysis (Pearce et al. 2020) of the images that Keralite transnational families share via social media offers insights into the discourse of elder abandonment, which is coupled with the negative discourse of migrants— and particularly migrating nurses—as exceptionally materialistic and individualistic people. These discourses are not only promoted through social media sites such as Facebook but also enter domestic spaces through more private chat applications like WhatsApp.

As Radhika Gajjala and Tarishi Verma (2018) described in their work on "WhatsAppified diasporas," the Indian women in their study perceived platforms such as Facebook, Twitter, and Instagram as public spaces in which they read information and post announcements intended for a wider audience, such as of births, deaths, and weddings. By contrast, the women used WhatsApp to express themselves more freely through chatting with friends and siblings, making this platform "a relational space for storing affective moments and sustaining transnational intimacies" (Gajjala and Verma 2018, 207). Memes shared in this way during the COVID-19 pandemic stirred discussions around what it means to be a good husband and wife (Narasimhan, Chittem, and Purang 2021). Similarly, when memes are shared within extended family groups of nurses via WhatsApp, they act as explicit reminders of what good eldercare entails and what it means to be a good daughter or son, no matter how far they might be from their homeland. In this way, social media and communication platforms contribute to the discourse of elder abandonment through international migration.

OLD AGE INSTITUTIONS

Besides migration, utilizing institutional eldercare is another way in which people may deviate from the ideal of intergenerational co-residence. In India, old age homes were founded through the efforts of Christian organizations during the British colonial era, with the first institution recorded as opening in 1882 in Kolkata, West Bengal (Lamb 2009, 57).[7] As Sarah Lamb (2009) has described, these homes were initially occupied almost exclusively by Anglo Indians of mixed English and Indian ancestry. Within their walls, the primary language was English, the clothing and food were predominantly European, and the most practiced religion was Christianity. All this contributed to the perception of the old age homes in India as grounded in Western rather than local— Hindu—ideologies of eldercare. To this day, people in India prefer to distance themselves from this 'Western habit' while proudly emphasizing "India's close-knit family culture" (Chadha 2020).[8]

The beliefs of Christians and Hindus about what good eldercare entails are grounded in distinct principles. Christians regard providing poor and aging people with a place to live as a service to them and thereby to God. By contrast, for Hindus, old age homes counter the principle of intergenerational co-residence, which is key to *sevā*, or service, that younger family members should provide to their aging relatives (Cohen 1998; Lamb 2000; Brijnath 2014). In a nutshell, *sevā* includes practices such as preparing and sharing food, offering tea, massaging feet, washing clothes, providing for medicines, and behaving respectfully toward

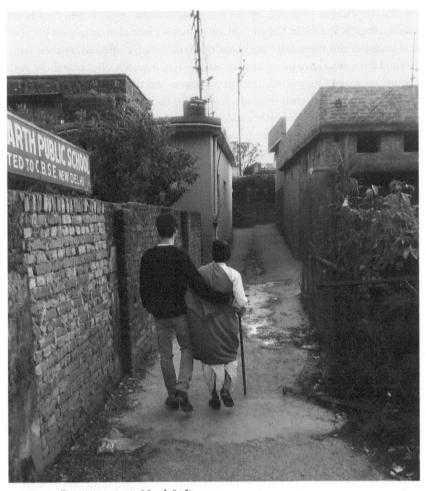

FIGURE 3.1. Practicing *sevā* in North India.

elders (figure 3.1). Now it also includes purchasing mobile phones, a practice that became a part of sevā along with the surge of international migration (Lamb 2009). In return, elders offer their blessings or, if they consider sevā poorly provided, curses. Sevā is integral to family relations of hierarchy, mutuality, and long-term deferred reciprocity, making it essentially tied to the household (Kowalski 2016; Brijnath 2014).[9]

In addition to aging Christians, the early old age homes historically provided accommodation and care to destitute locals who had no family, whose closest family members had predeceased them, or whose family members could not provide care because of poverty. The association of old age homes with categories such as old, poor, and female persisted through the 1990s (Cohen 1998, 117; Lamb 2000), and it was still going strong during my fieldwork. As noted in the *Manual on Old Age Homes*, prepared by the nongovernmental organization Centre for Gerontological Studies in Kerala, "old age homes are intended mainly for the poor and indigent and those who are abandoned/deserted/neglected by their families and those who have no other place to go" (Nayar 2016, 2). Because these institutions are mainly supported through donations and the goodwill of those who run them, there are no clear regulations regarding the qualifications of the carers or the appropriateness of spaces for residents who might have special needs. The persisting negative views of old age homes emanate from, and reinforce, the ideal of intergenerational co-residence. A large majority of older people in India remain convinced that their children should take care of them financially, physically, and emotionally (James et al. 2013, 42; see also De Jong 2011, 2014).

Yet at the same time aged-care homes have recently mushroomed around the country, especially in the major urban centers (Lamb 2009). Although the first old age homes were founded in Kerala only in 1957, estimates suggest that this state has the highest number of these institutions in India, with a 69 percent increase between 2011 and 2015 (Augustine, George, and Sudhir Kumar 2020).[10] Through my fieldwork I discovered that these institutions come in many shapes and sizes: from old age shelters or orphanages to geriatric hospitals and—a recent development—luxurious residencies. The differences between them are tied to social class; shelters are most similar to the earlier old age homes described by Lamb (2000) and Cohen (1998).

Contemporary old age homes have developed to attend to a broader clientele, including those from the middle classes whose children or other relatives are working abroad. In what follows, I show how money shapes the (perceived) degree of the residents' agency, and how this in turn influences whether they are enacted as abandoned or agentive residents of eldercare institutions.

OLD AGE SHELTERS

At 7:00 A.M. the traffic in Kottayam was already busy, and the freshness of the early morning was blending with the heaviness of fumes and noise. I was sitting in a car next to Veena, who had come to pick me up before breakfast. She and her mother Suncy had invited me to join them on their visit to a local old age shelter, which was run by a Christian church. It was Suncy's husband's death anniversary, and such an event is usually commemorated in Kerala by doing a good deed for those in need. For this purpose, Suncy wanted to donate some food and clothes to the women living in the shelter, so she had risen at 4:00 A.M. to cook while Veena prepared a bag of secondhand saris. As the gently crisp air was stroking my face through the open car window, I asked her to tell me more about the kind of people who lived in the shelter. They were, she said without hesitation, people "discarded by their family, abandoned, they have no one, or they are widows."

We arrived at the shelter at 7:10 A.M., ten minutes late. Everyone was up and waiting for us. One of the nuns, whom Veena called "Sister," greeted us at the entrance of the compound. The courtyard as well as the buildings were clean and neat, quite unlike what I had imagined given the popular and academic accounts of these places as decrepit and grubby. The floor was freshly mopped, and the wooden tables in the dining room were protected with clear vinyl covers and flanked by red plastic chairs. One table was covered with a beautiful green table-cloth and was set with glass cups and porcelain plates. This, obviously, was the table for the guests of honor.

While Suncy and Veena were occupied setting out food on the main table for self-service, one of the nuns took me around. She showed me some of the simple but clean shared rooms where the women stayed, and she said that they were providing accommodation for seventeen women and had the capacity for another three. As we sat on a wooden bench on the shaded terrace and looked at the courtyard, lit with soft sunlight, the nun explained to me that the shelter was run by three Christian nuns and one assistant, all women. The residents were over the age of 60 and were generally healthy, but one had mental health problems, and two others needed assistance with activities of daily living such as with eating and bathing. Most were Christian, although a few were Hindu or Muslim. Regardless of their religious background, they were all expected to attend the Christian mass held every morning in the chapel in the compound.

Anita, the sister in charge, told me this was a place for poor people and "orphans." Families with children who were nurses were not poor, and they would rather place their aging parents in old age homes, she said. In this shelter, only 70-year-old Manju had a daughter who worked as a nurse in the Gulf. Anita briefly summarized Manju's story to me. After her second child died, Manju's hus-band became abusive to her, and she finally divorced him. He was a drunkard, Manju reportedly claimed.

As I sat on the bench listening to Alice's recount, Manju was right there in front of us, wearing a bright pink flowery nightie and sweeping the floor. She had noticed that we were talking about her, and she approached but did not sit next to us. Still holding the broom, she began telling her story in Malayalam, with tears in her eyes and loudly enough for anyone around to hear. After her divorce, Manju's daughter stayed with her father because Manju had no income. Manju moved in with one of her male relatives as a maid, but that situation was fraught as well. She eventually decided to move to the old age shelter. I asked her, through Anita, to tell us more about how she had made the decision to move. Manju frowned, waved her hand, and left.

By way of explaining Manju's behavior, Anita said that there was some "tension, depression." She concluded, "Well, anyway, that's the story that she's telling." Suncy, who had joined us toward the end of the conversation with Manju, knowingly nodded. But I was confused: what was this supposed to mean? "Oh, maybe it's all lies," Suncy replied, ending the discussion.

OLD AGE HOMES

As places where people could live rather than just visit occasionally, old age shelters, old age homes, and geriatric hospitals challenge the ideals and realities of
co-residence and other kinship-based principles of filial reciprocity. In Kerala,
these institutions have very different reputations, and this is importantly tied to
money. Old age shelters are free of charge, while old age homes and geriatric
hospitals generally charge fees. People often used the terms home and shelter
interchangeably when the particular institution they were referring to had both a
"pay-for-stay" and a free section.

This was the case at the old age home run by the Mundakapadam Mandirams
Society, which catered to clients of different socioeconomic backgrounds.[11]
For "the well-to-do," their website advertised three types of apartments for
rent, from 400-square-foot one-bedroom apartments to 800-square-foot two-
bedroom apartments. The prospective resident had to make a deposit of 6 to
14 *lahks* (about USD 8,100–19,000), depending on the accommodation type. Each
year, the organization deducted 10 percent of this deposit as a rent payment.[12] In
addition, residents paid INR 5,600 (about USD 80) monthly for food and estab-
lishment charges. By contrast, the Mandirams Society website described the free
section for older adults, called Aghati Mandiram, as the "Poor Home for the aged,
sick, penniless and abandoned men and women . . . who had once borne the
neglect of their near and dear ones."[13]

One morning in March 2015, I caught a clunky yellow rickshaw taxi to take me
to the Mandirams Society compound. I found myself standing in front of a cluster
of peach-colored buildings, including a church, soaking in the serenity of the surrounding greenery, which was in stark contrast to the boisterous streets of Kottayam. I approached the main office door, and I left my flip-flops next to a line of
men's slippers on the brown marble stairs. Once inside, the secretary asked me to
write a formal letter about the intention of my visit. Then I was briskly introduced
to a young woman who volunteered at the institution and was designated as my
guide.

She first led me to the section where the residents paid a fee to live in small
apartments. The first older woman we encountered had children abroad, but
none of them were nurses; she directed us toward another apartment to meet
Susan, who was a retired nurse and teacher herself. Susan took the opportunity
of my visit as a break from watching television. Kerala had been brewing with
political tensions that would result the next day in a *hartal*—roadblocks and the
complete closure of shops and services to protest the government. Susan, a sharp
woman in her 70s with short gray hair, was wearing a blue-and-white nightie; her
English was impeccable. She said that her father had initially disapproved of the
nursing profession, but Susan and three of her four sisters eventually became
nurses. Two of them worked in the United States, and the third one worked in

Kuwait. Susan's own children did not continue the profession, but they did migrate abroad. Her son lived in Dubai and her daughter in the United States; they both provided the money for her rent, and they called her daily on the phone, she told us.

I was surprised to learn that Susan did not live alone in the apartment. A young woman from Tamil Nadu, small and lean, stayed with her as her maid. While her maid made tea for us in the kitchenette, separate from the living room, Susan explained that the girl had been studying nursing but had to suspend her studies because she could not pay the tuition fees. If she decided to continue her studies, Susan would "support" her, she told me. Through co-residence, the relationship between Susan and her maid came to be one of "fictive kinship" (Karner 1998; see also Brijnath 2009). In this case, care was mediated through money in the form of salary and the potential of student fees. Money therefore contributed to mutual care, even as the relationship between two women remained asymmetric, given the class and age differences between them.[14]

Susan had moved into the old age home voluntarily a couple of years earlier because she did not want to live alone in her ancestral home after her husband's death. That house was in a semirural area, too remote for an older woman to live alone or to attract a maid. Susan asserted that living at an old age home was "heaven" for her, although she recognized that some people thought it was "hell." But those people "only knew about the other part of it, the orphanage," she explained. She enjoyed the place because all its facilities were available to her—a doctor and nurse visited each week for an extra fee of INR 50 (less than USD 1) or so, and if Susan needed something she could call her maid or somebody from the church.[15] Even prayer was transmitted through loudspeakers, so she did not have to walk across the courtyard to the church. Instead, she could attend the mass by simply sitting on the terrace in front of her apartment.

Every day at 5:00 P.M., five of Susan's friends from the compound strolled over to her veranda for tea and talk. Susan's lunch and dinner were delivered daily from the canteen, and she could enjoy them in the privacy of her apartment. Unlike some other residents of the pay-for-stay compound, Susan did not mind that her food was prepared in the same kitchen as the food for "the orphans."

My visit with the Mandirams Society continued in the canteen where the so-called orphans—the residents of the old age shelter, "the orphanage"—were having their lunch (figure 3.2). The atmosphere was not as cheerful as in Susan's apartment. The people who bent their heads over their plates were thin and had the darker complexions so commonly associated in India with lower classes and castes; some were disabled, and all were quiet and looked serious.[16] There were about thirty residents in this shelter, and about half of them were men. The young woman who was accompanying me asked me to sit at a table for lunch next to two well-dressed, corpulent women who clearly did not live there. They were visitors: the younger had brought food for the orphans for the Remembrance Day for her

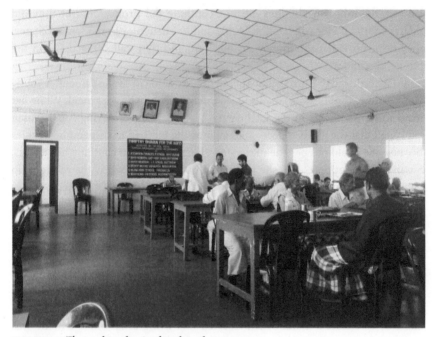

FIGURE 3.2. The orphans having lunch in the canteen.

father, just as Veena and Suncy had done. There was a prayer, during which every-one sat silently, but some did not care much about it and started eating well before the prayer ended.

So even within the same institution that provided services to aging people, different sections could be markedly different based on who they were catering to in terms of their socioeconomic status. Many residents in the pay-for-stay section of the Mandirams Society had children abroad; other similar institutions hosted people from different family situations.

A "charitable trust" run by another church in Kottayam rented rooms exclu-sively to older women at INR 1,500 (about USD 23) monthly, plus a security deposit. At the time of my visit, seven women lived there, and a few rooms—small apartments with attached bathrooms—were still available. Thresiamma, the bishop's wife who oversaw the home, explained to me that women who wanted to stay there had to be recommended by their parish or *panchayat* (vil-lage council), and their relatives were asked to provide their contact details and "be responsible." This meant that the family had to finance their relative's stay and promise that they would accommodate her in the event she no longer could take care of herself due to physical or mental decline. Residents in this pay-for-stay home had to do their own washing and cooking, or they could buy their food in a canteen. There was no doctor on the premises, but the management would help arrange a visit for the residents if needed. At first Thresiamma told me that women preferred to live in a community like theirs rather than alone because of safety. But then, as we were walking slowly down the hall greeting one resident after another, an administrator happened to pass by who noted that three of the women staying there were not married, one was separated, and another three were widows—and all of them had children who lived nearby.

"If they have children but stay here, it's because of this . . ." Thresiamma made a gesture with her hands, crossing her index fingers in the air. "Family disputes. These are well-to-do-women, their families have the money to pay for the rent, but they don't want to live with their daughters-in-law."

Thresiamma's comment reminded me of Manju, the lady I had met at the shelter for women that I described earlier. As ethnographic accounts from other parts of India show, family conflicts are a "common source of affliction facing people in old age" (Lamb 2000, 71). The relationship between the mother-in-law and daughter-in-law may be especially fraught with tension because they are both bonded to the same male person whose attention and affection they antici-pate and strive for (Lamb 2000; Trawick 1990). Despite any conflicts that may arise, however, the ideal would be for the family to solve it without anyone of their elders moving out of their ancestral home.

GERIATRIC HOSPITALS

There were very few geriatric hospitals in the area where I was staying; I heard only about a couple of them and visited one in person. Established in 1949 by a Protestant priest, the Fellowship Hospital in Kumbarad opened its geriatric ward in 2007. When I visited it in 2014, eighty-three patients—thirteen men and seventy women—were staying there. I met most of them as I went on a morning round with Siju, a young, energetic female doctor, who sported black, broad-rimmed glasses and a white coat, respectively signaling her commitment to pro-gress and medical professionalism. She told me that, given their poor health, the ward residents were unlikely to ever leave. In this sense, the ward was a sort of hospice, providing palliative care to bedridden people.

The ages of the resident-patients ranged from 57 to "about 100 years," Siju explained to me. She was quick to add that people brought their relatives to the ward "more easily than to other eldercare institutions because there is the hospi-tal nearby." This allowed for good care in terms of consistent medical attention, and Siju provided an example. Recently, one of the patients had hurt her head and became dizzy, so Siju wanted to administer an X-ray scan of her brain. To do that, she first had to call the patient's family and ask their permission, and only then could the patient be taken to the main hospital in the neighboring building for the scan.

My friend Madesh interpreted Siju's statement as implying that the geriatric hospital had a better reputation than old age homes and shelters for two reasons.

First, residents had to pay for their accommodation and care; furthermore, the hospital was associated with clinical services. As the example of the X-ray scan indicates, care in the hospital related to attending to the body and physical health, provided that the resident-patient's family agreed to—and would pay for—the medical treatments. A place in the geriatric hospital cost INR 15,000 (about USD 230) per month, and nursing and medical services costs added another INR 15,000 or so to the bill.[17]

Families could also choose to pay for an extra service: several patients I met had a woman sitting next to them to chat and attend to any needs they might have. These women "companions" spent time with patients most days of the week, from early morning to 5:00 in the afternoon. As the head nurse explained to me, all residents had at least one relative working abroad who covered these expenses. None, however, had a child who was working abroad as a nurse.

THE ABANDONED AND THE AGENTIVE

The old age shelters that I visited in Kerala were very much in line with Lawrence Cohen's (1998) description of such places decades earlier in Varanasi, a city in the northern Indian state of Uttar Pradesh. Most strikingly, little, if any, agency was attributed to the aging residents. As one of my interlocutors told me, "the children who leave their parents in shelters don't work abroad; they just don't care for them." It thus makes sense that these institutions were also referred to as "orphanages" and their residents as "orphans." The word orphan was used to refer to any person with no immediate family, either in the generation above or below. At the same time, this word might also imply that the residents were considered as children—helpless and without family members who would cater to their very basic needs, such as providing them with food and a roof over their heads.

Yet the old age shelters I encountered also contained stories that were told less from the standpoint of victimhood and more of agency (see also Lamb 2000). One female resident of the women's shelter in Kottayam, Amma, was exceptionally keen to talk to me. She called one of the sisters who worked there to act as a translator for us. Amma introduced herself as a widow with three daughters. After her husband's death, her daughters had to decide how to organize care for their mother and, specifically, how to arrange where she would live. Finally, they told her that she would have to move from one daughter's household to another's every two weeks because their husbands did not want her to stay in their homes permanently (see chapter 5). Amma considered this and then decided to move to the shelter voluntarily for her own peace of mind and stability. She enjoyed living there, and she was very active, especially in taking care of the shelter garden.

The general discourse of eldercare institutions in Kerala is based on the assumption that those who pay for their stay in old age homes have more agency

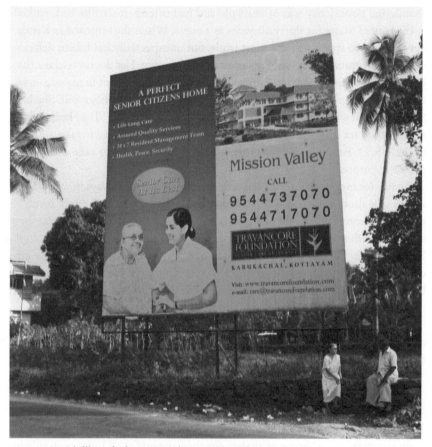

FIGURE 3.3. A billboard advertising a luxury old age home.

than those receiving free residence.[18] Pay-for-stay homes are considered in a more positive light as places where aging people can find company, especially if their children have migrated abroad or if they are returning migrants themselves. Targeting this specific audience, an upgraded version of these homes as luxurious "assisted living communities" (figure 3.3) has been proliferating across Kerala in recent years (e.g., Vishwanathan 2013).[19] With some variation, residents of old age shelters, paid old age homes, and geriatric hospitals were commonly enacted as either "abandoned" or "agentive" depending on their socioeconomic class and, consequently, the type of institution they could afford to live in. In this way, money contributed to enacting better-off older adults as people with higher autonomy and self-determination than those who with more limited financial resources.[20]

However, in the geriatric hospital I came across one person whose experience defied clear distinction along the lines of the agentive affluent people and the abandoned poor. Jancy was 63 years old and had osteoporosis. She had worked in the United States for thirty-six years as a nurse. When she returned to Kerala, her plan was to stay only for a short while, but unexpectedly her health deteriorated, and eventually she could not even sit up anymore. Her doctor told me that Jancy had decided herself to come to the geriatric hospital, but in my conversation with her Jancy insisted she had been placed there against her will. She had two sons, each with his own family, living in the United States. "They keep telling me that they are sorry," she explained, "but they have never tried to take me back to the US. . . . People today are more selfish; nobody wants to take care of old people anymore."

I have not met her sons, so I can only imagine the various ways in which they would talk about their mother's situation and their own lack of direct involvement in her care. Perhaps they had financial problems themselves, or maybe they struggled with pressure at work and worried about the future of their children. Did they truly not care? Or were they so overwhelmed with their own life circumstances to be unable to do more for their mother? What was the relationship between the mother and each of the two sons, and how had this unfolded over the years?

I have no answers to these questions. But it seems that the discourse of elder abandonment may also serve to elicit sympathy for the parent and act as an emotional remedy in some situations.

LIVING ALONE, FEELING ALONE

The question of whether children will actually fulfill their filial obligations is an open question and a source of anxiety for their parents at all times, not only in cases of international migration (Vatuk 1990, 84). I came across stories in personal conversations, in the press, and in scholarly writings that served as warnings: most prominently, parents should never sign official documents to transfer property rights to their children before death; otherwise, their children might take their home and land while ignoring filial obligations. In other words, the dread that children will default on their obligations and become ungrateful, greedy adults who abandon their parents as soon as they have access to their inheritance is ever present (Muruvelil 2015; Sebastian and Sekher 2018).

Such accounts represented the grounds for the Maintenance and Welfare of Parents and Senior Citizens Bill, inaugurated by the Indian Parliament in 2007, which has instituted eldercare not only as a moral but also a legal obligation (Lamb 2009, 237–238). In 2018, the Kerala state government announced that it would become stricter in implementing this bill because the number of people who had children but lived in government-run old age homes had been increasing among low- and middle-class families (Chandran 2018). Interestingly, although the people I met and the press regularly questioned the quality of care provided in old age homes, the quality of care at family homes was rarely doubted. There seemed to be few mechanisms to monitor family-provided care other than through occasional visits from attentive neighbors, friends, and acquaintances.[21]

How does intergenerational co-residence translate into good eldercare? A partial answer to this question may be offered by the following account in which an Ayurvedic doctor contrasted the situations of two older men.

First, as an example of the limits to the ideal of co-residence, the doctor told me about one of his patients, a widower living with his married son. This man's son and daughter-in-law both worked, and the grandchildren were in school all day. In the evening, the son would ask his father if he had eaten; he would reply yes, and that was it—no further conversation ensued. Because providing food and co-residence are basic care practices in India, the son appeared to consider this question to be sufficient fulfillment of his care duties toward his father. Deprived of everyday social contacts, the older man would go to the nearby bus stop every day just to sit and watch people walk by. In the evening, he would return home.

The doctor continued by recounting the story of another male patient, an 80-year-old widower whose children were abroad. He lived alone and had "lots of health problems." The doctor suggested that he find a paying guest to help in case of emergency. But the man replied that his son returned home every year for one month, and so he wanted to keep the room empty for him. If the room were rented out, where would his son stay? "Because this man wants his son to live with him for one month per year," the doctor continued, "he suffers for eleven other months."

These two men, the doctor concluded, had the same problem: loneliness. One lived completely alone and the other with his son, but the latter was lonely nonetheless because his family members were busy with their own lives. The doctor concluded that many older adults came to see him just to chat, and that was why he took time to talk to them.

The story of these two old men and their loneliness reminded me of another older man I had met. One evening, Meera, a middle-aged married woman who was completing her PhD studies in biology, invited me to have dinner with her family. Through chance encounters at an Ayurvedic clinic where I had briefly stayed we became friendly, and I also came to know her husband and teenage daughter. Once I entered the kitchen at her home and, to my surprise, I noticed that Meera was making only the chapattis herself—all the curries she had bought "somewhere else." The fact that Meera was buying food outside rather than cooking it—and that she was shy about it—is indicative of the struggles that contemporary women in India experience as they try to combine their professional careers with the ideal of being a good wife, mother, and daughter-in-law (see also Narasimhan, Chittem, and Purang 2021). Indeed, besides migration, some people in India regard the increasing professional education of women and their

60

entering into the workforce as another significant danger to good eldercare (Jamuna 2003; Shankardass and Rajan 2018).

In the dining room, Meera's husband and daughter were watching an Asian movie awards program on television with the sound up loud. I sat down at the dining table, and eventually Meera's father-in-law joined us, sliding quietly through the room. Nobody acknowledged his presence. "Good evening," I said to him, but he did not reply—perhaps he had not heard me. Meera's husband told him, smiling, that I had greeted him, and the old man turned to me and mumbled, "Good evening." Meera served us food, but instead of joining us at the table she hurried back into the kitchen. To my surprise, throughout dinner there was no talk at all; all eyes were glued to the television screen.

Was the silence among the family members with whom I shared a meal a sign of profound intimacy, in which exchanging words was less important, or a sort of intergenerational disconnection? The answer might be somewhere in between and subject to change at any given time. The stories I have described in this chapter all demonstrate that it is difficult to make assumptions about elder abandonment, especially in relation to loneliness and isolation. People may feel lonely at any age, despite having rich social contacts or even living with their children (Lamb 2009, 181; Von Faber and van der Geest 2010). Because of complex personal relations, family histories, and other circumstances, living alone—just like living together with family members—may involve loneliness and invoke a plethora of other emotions.

Most of all, that evening with Meera's family, along with the Ayurvedic doctor's stories, made clear to me that distance is about more than geography or location. Physical proximity and meeting filial obligations through co-residence does not automatically translate into emotional closeness or lively social interaction. In the second part of this book, I show how transnational families have reconceptualized migration from an act of abandonment into a care practice, a transformation in which digital technologies and remittances have played a key role.

PART 2 CARING THROUGH TRANSNATIONAL COLLECTIVES

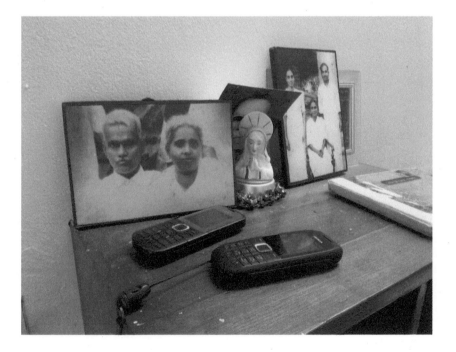

4 · CALLING FREQUENTLY

In October 2014, I found myself writing notes on my laptop at a wooden kitchen table in Margaret's apartment in Hilia, a middle-sized desert town in Oman.[1] Margaret was a nurse in her 50s who lived by herself, while her three teenage children stayed with her husband and father-in-law in Kerala. Next to me, sunk into an old, soft couch was Ashu, Margaret's peer and friend, completely absorbed in her smartphone. This was how she was keeping me company while Margaret was at work. During the weeks of my stay, Ashu often dropped by, even if only to sit next to an electrical socket, plug in her smartphone, and keep her eyes glued to the screen for hours. She scrolled through Facebook and typed messages to her family members and friends in other countries in silence. "Margaret's Wi-Fi is much better than mine," she would say by way of explaining herself.

The apartment that Margaret rented was a spacious, spotlessly clean, and scantily furnished two-bedroom apartment above a series of small shops and eateries, just behind a petrol station. She paid 80 Omani rial (about 200 US dollars) per month for her rent; her monthly salary was OMR 900 (USD 2,340). She knew many of her colleagues shared a house to bring the rent down to OMR 30 per person (USD 80), but she did not like the idea of sharing a residence. In this way, family members could visit her at any time without having to adjust to any non-kin roommates.

Many of the items in her apartment, including the furniture, towels, and bedsheets, were provided for by the Omani Ministry of Health through a one-time compensation of OMR 2,000 (USD 5,000). The austere look of Margaret's residence was not a consequence of poverty but devotion: this was how she chose to express her commitment to God. For the same reason she also mopped the red-tiled ceramic floor twice daily, and she always—even when visiting others' houses—sat and slept on the floor. Small, stout, and wearing rimless glasses, Margaret dressed in unobtrusive beige *salwari kurtas* or even denim shirts, and I never saw her in a sari.

Margaret's appearance and attitude were in stark contrast to Ashu's, who was the social one among them. Ashu's bright-pink *salwar kameez* fluttered as she

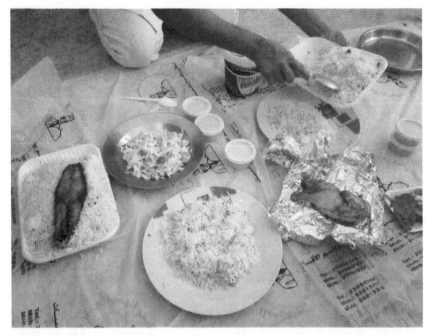

FIGURE 4.1. Serving dinner.

scurried from having a chat with the Muslim girl next door to catching the bus that would take her—and once also me—to the United Arab Emirates (UAE) to see her sister, which she did every weekend when she was off duty.

During my stay Margaret and Ashu both took care of me jointly, bringing *dosa*, a thin crepe accompanied by savory curries, for breakfast and chicken with rice for dinner, which they would serve on a plastic sheet spread on the floor next to the table (figure 4.1). Because it was so convenient to buy ready-made food from nearby takeouts, they rarely cooked for themselves.

In their polyclinic, where they enjoyed a comfortable work schedule from 7:00 A.M. to 2:30 P.M. with no night shifts—which was quite different from India, where shifts could spread from 8:00 A.M. to 6:00 P.M.—Margaret and Ashu had joined forces with about fifteen Indian, fifteen Omani, and thirty or forty Filipino nurses, and they introduced me to several of them. On my very first day, we visited a house that hosted four Indian families who split the rent, and then several single-family households where nurses—some pregnant—lived with their husbands and small children. A Bangladeshi female doctor hosted a dinner party for us at her home, decorated with ornate vases, glass statues, and thick wood furniture, all too lavish for Margaret's taste. Together, the Indian and Filipino nurses often celebrated holidays, birthdays, and transitions to other countries.

Socializing with Omanis, however, happened on extremely rare occasions, such as hosting a Westerner like myself. Upon hearing about me, two Omani hospital "directors" eagerly volunteered to take us for several outings in the surrounding area. One of these excursions included an afternoon trip to the local market. There, a party of two senior Indian women and two middle-aged Omani men accompanying a young Western woman was quite a sight for the Muslim fruit sellers from Kerala. In fact, they were so pleasantly surprised to encounter their compatriots that they refused to charge for the watermelons that Margaret and Ashu wanted to purchase and offered the fruit as a gift. In the six years of residing in Hillia, the two women had never come close to the market. The Indian nurses' physical movements, it transpired, were limited to their workplace, their residence, and occasionally their colleagues' homes. This reflected their social movements as well, which were restricted to their circle of Asian migrant co-workers and strictly separated from the local population.

But as Ashu's intense involvement with her smartphone indicated, nurses in Oman frequently socialized in another way—through digital technologies. The way in which Ashu engaged with her smartphone, often and intensely, was more of a rule than an exception. One evening, Margaret and Ashu invited over a co-worker to paint my hands with *mehendi*, the brown paste of the henna plant used in India to draw magnificent, temporary tattoos for festivities such as marriage and sometimes just for fun. Along came Benny, a lean, dark-skinned laboratory technician with a short moustache, and his very pregnant wife, a nurse. He started recounting his own experience of using the mobile phone to keep in touch with his mother who lived alone in Kerala. Unable to take notes while the paint was still drying on my fingers, I struggled to memorize his account, which was so surprising that it easily stuck with me. Benny told me that when he first moved to Oman in 2007, he called his mother fifteen to twenty times a day, and sometimes more often than that. At the time, he was posted in an isolated small village. Later, after he had relocated to Hillia and his wife joined him, he reduced the number of calls, but he still talked to his mother four or five times every day. Although the frequency of Benny's calls was remarkable, most migrating nurses in other families also called their parents living in Kerala at least once a day.

Talking regularly, even daily on the phone to one's parents clearly "mattered" (Miller 1998) to the nurses who had migrated abroad, but how? What did they try to achieve through this practice? And given their prominent role in the everyday life of transnational families, how did digital technologies influence how family members related to one another?

In chapter 1, I introduced material semiotics and argued that this theoretical approach is fruitful for exploring the subtle impacts of digital technologies on transnational families. In this chapter, I describe in detail how the people in such families and their digital technologies create transnational care collectives, how they enact care through these collectives, and how they determine how such care should be done to be considered good. I then explore how care is not only directed toward aging parents but becomes distributed among all the members of the collective, human and nonhuman. Finally, I investigate how different types of technologies shape different modes of relating among transnational family members.

TRANSNATIONAL CARE COLLECTIVES

Transnational care collectives are assemblages of human and nonhuman actors that participate in certain practices through which care becomes enacted across geographic distance (see also chapter 1). These collectives primarily include adult children who migrate abroad, their parents who remain in their homeland, and the digital technologies that they use to reach each other. Through tinkering, each transnational care collective establishes its own dynamic, depending on which types of digital technologies become included, who calls whom and how often, and how the collective is expanded to people beyond the parent–child(ren) dyad.

Tinkering with Digital Technologies

One evening in Kottayam, while waiting for her mother to prepare dinner, Mary, a young unmarried nurse still living with her parents, proudly showed me her collection of four mobile phones. Two of them were simple mobile phones; the other two were smartphones. All four devices had been bought as gifts by Mary's sisters, who worked in the United Kingdom. When I asked Mary why she kept them all, she replied, "To show them to my nephews one day, so they will know how well my sisters took care of us!"

Mary's parents each had their own basic mobile phone, similar to those in figure 4.2, and additionally the family had a laptop with a USB webcam. Their house was equipped with a landline phone and wireless internet for which the family paid about INR 300 (around USD 4) per month for unlimited use. All their devices and subscriptions to the landline phone and the internet were provided and paid for by the two daughters who lived abroad.

The presence of so many digital technologies was quite typical of the families I encountered. Mobile phones, smartphones, personal computers, laptops, and tablets were commonly provided by the migrating children, who also paid for the telecommunication services needed to use them. These devices were more than just gifts—they served to create transnational care collectives.

When I started my fieldwork in 2014, mobile phones were most common type of technology used by older adults. Text-based forms of communication such as smart message service (SMS) or internet-based messenger services like WhatsApp were more popular among siblings and the younger members of transnational families. Email, by contrast, was reserved for official communications, such as sending documents. Indeed, only one nurse in Oman told me that she had emailed her parents once to send them some legal documents.[2] To communicate with their parents, adult children preferred to rely on phone calls.

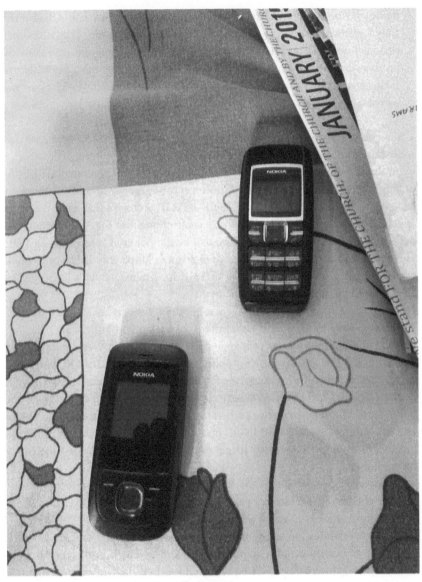

FIGURE 4.2. Simple phones, bought and inherited.

Looking at me from the screen during one of our first Skype conversations, Anthony, a nurse who first had worked in the United Kingdom and then Australia, described how and why he preferred calling his parents on the phone over using any other digital technology:

It's not that expensive to call to India from Australia. I don't have a subscription; I have a prepaid mobile phone. It costs 2 cents [USD 0.01] per minute to call home, and the connection rate is about 29 cents [USD 0.21] per call. In the United Kingdom there was no connection charge; it was only 1 pence [USD 0.01] per minute. I don't use the internet to call my parents. Sometimes I use it to call my brother and friends who use similar apps, but my parents don't normally use them. But really, I don't mind spending 2 cents per minute to speak to my parents.

Calling on the phone was therefore favored because it was free or inexpensive as well as the most practical for the parents.

Anthony was aware of "Voice over Internet Protocol" (VoIP) service, a free technology that enables audio calls over the internet to any mobile or landline phone. In fact, Skype is just one among many kinds of VoIP protocols that are available as applications to download on laptop or a smartphone. But for Anthony, prepaid mobile phone calls were so inexpensive that he did not even consider using VoIP. He preferred to pay these small amounts to adapt to his parents' habits of technology use. If he wanted them to switch to VoIP, his parents would have needed to acquire smartphones and the skills to use them.

In a polymedia environment where a number of media coexist and are constantly evaluated in relation to each other (Madianou and Miller 2012), flexibility and pragmatism in terms of convenience, rather than cost, were key for nurses like Anthony. This reflected the economic situation of their families, which had usually improved following migration (Percot 2014). At the same time, the availability of digital technologies greatly depended on the country in which the nurses lived. Those in countries such as the United Kingdom, the United States, and Australia often used VoIP to call on mobile and landline phones in Kerala, but this technology was mostly illegal in the Gulf countries at the time of my research there.

Some have speculated that the VoIP ban was enforced to protect the revenues of the national telecom operators (Aziz 2012), but the Omani Telecom Regulatory Authority maintained that the decision to only allow VoIP through local telecommunication operators was based on security concerns (Nair 2016). To add to the confusion, the regulations regarding which VoIP services were considered legal were changed frequently and sometimes without much public notice. In 2012, for example, Google Talk, Viber, FaceTime, and MSN Messenger were suddenly made available while Skype remained blocked (ITP Staff 2012).

Most nurses thus navigated several VoIP services interchangeably, trying to follow the law to the best of their knowledge. For example, Benny, the laboratory technician I met in Oman at our little *mehendi* party, used calling applications such as Rounds, Imo, MoSIP (he used this one to call his mother daily because "the sound was clear"), Facebook Messenger, Talkray ("often busy"), and Viber before it became banned. When I started noting down this list of calling applications, Benny's face suddenly froze with fear: if any of these apps happened to be illegal at that moment, would talking to me get him into trouble? After all, he had just met me briefly through a work colleague and was not sure of my intentions. I managed to calm him down, but his reaction threw light on another issue: the rules about VoIP changed so quickly that it was difficult to be sure which digital technologies were allowed at any given moment. Yet breaking them could lead to serious trouble: in 2009, the police raided internet cafés throughout the country and arrested over 200 people of various Asian nationalities for facilitating VoIP (Metz 2009).

Technologies "never stand alone, because they must always be connected with existing infrastructures" (Jensen and Winthereik 2013, 5). Although seemingly unbounded, digital technologies are embedded in their local physical as well as sociopolitical environment, including its infrastructure, which supports or limits how they work. Digital technologies need the infrastructure of the electrical grid for power and the telecommunication infrastructure to establish a connection between phones, smartphones, or laptops. These infrastructures could be described as "absent presence" (Law 2002): they are essential for digital technologies to function, yet they are generally invisible to end users—if not always physically, then at least in terms of how much attention people pay to them when they are chatting on the phone and responding to messages on social media. Furthermore, like technologies, infrastructures are not universal; they differ from one location to another, and they are subject to the regional forces of nature and to local communities at various scales (Edwards 2003).

By extension, transnational care collectives depend on how digital technologies are locally situated within these infrastructures and communities. Just as infrastructures support collectives, they may also disrupt or limit them, so "the inability of technologies to perform their functions must be subject to the same critical scrutiny as their achievements" (Larkin 2008, 219). Technological breakdowns of infrastructure impact the functioning of digital technologies—for example, through poor connectivity, low credit on the phone or internet prepaid card, or the interruption of the electricity supply due to weather events. Disruptions like these reflect the government's capacity to maintain telecommunication and other related services and to repair and quickly re-establish connections in case of load shedding, brownouts, and burnouts. Such breakdowns, or "interferences" (Pype 2018), may occur more commonly in some countries than in others, making transnational care collectives relatively easier or more difficult to create based on the geographic locations in which they are grounded.

Transnational care collectives with family members in Oman were clearly influenced by the local sociopolitical and economic forces that supported certain infrastructures and limited others, which guided the availability of VoIP calling applications. These circumstances were also subject to various changes through time. The impact of the COVID-19 pandemic indicated one such influence.

At that time, in 2020, several human rights organizations called on the Gulf countries to unblock VoIP for video and audio calls to enable migrant workers of all nationalities to communicate with their families overseas (Human Rights Watch 2020). In response to these "exceptional circumstances," Oman lifted the ban on Skype, Google Meet, and Zoom, with the primary aim to facilitate communication in business and government institutions (Yousuf 2020).

Transnational care collectives are also continuously reshaped through relatively rapid innovation and uptake of new digital technologies. During my fieldwork in 2014–2015, digital devices that enabled the transmission of visual images were used less commonly than simple mobile and landline phones. This trend has been shifting over the past several years, especially since the spread of WhatsApp—which has earned India the nickname of "the WhatsApp nation" (Sengupta 2021). According to the *Telegraph India*, a daily newspaper in English, 400 million people in India had downloaded WhatsApp by 2021 (Sengupta 2021; see also Jain 2021). In my follow-up interviews between 2018 and 2022, several people told me that Skype was "a thing of the past" because it had been replaced by WhatsApp, a commercial-free application developed for smartphones. Compared with Skype, which was initially designed to support voice calls from one personal computer to another, WhatsApp is much easier to use for everyone, including older adults (Cowling 2016; Pahwa 2021).

In 2021, a comparison of these two platforms came up during a conversation I had with Anthony. Because we met online, no food was shared, as had been the custom whenever I visited people in Kerala, and the only impression of his home I got was of a dark sofa leaning against an empty white wall. But what he told me about the developments in his transnational care collective was fascinating:

> My grandmother is 95 years old now, and my mother is 61, they live together in Kerala. I call them every day, recently mostly on WhatsApp. When I spoke to you six years ago, my parents were not comfortable handling smartphones at all. But since then, everyone got a smartphone, and everyone has become comfortable with using applications like WhatsApp or Facebook. I'm not saying that my mother is proficient in all smartphone apps, but she can contact people through a video call on WhatsApp. I think the use of Skype has been gradually reducing over the last years in India since WhatsApp is easier to use. We still have Skype for official purposes—we use it at work—but otherwise it's very rare.

Tinkering is about attentive experimenting, trying out the various choices, and making adjustments in care relations to find out which practices, situations, and settings are the most suitable for all those involved in a care collective. It is the normative and creative "process of caring by adapting to changing situations" (Pols 2012, 166). Family members have thus tinkered with various digital devices and software communication programs until they found what suited them best, at least until they found something better. The choice of specific digital technologies usually depended on the parents' skills and comfort regarding the technologies as well as telecommunication availability and reliability in different countries.

The stories of people I met highlighted their constant tinkering with digital devices, people's knowledge and abilities, preferences and possibilities—including in terms of telecommunication infrastructures shaped by their sociopolitical circumstances—to establish the best possible way of sustaining transnational care collectives.

Beyond Parents and Children

Devices that afforded the production and sharing of images (either photographs or short video clips) or enabled video calls were particularly useful in expanding the transnational care collective to other kin and non-kin members. Most often, they included migrating nurses' own children or siblings who still lived with their parents in Kerala. In 2014–2015, before the widespread use of WhatsApp, webcam calling was typically conducted through Skype or Facebook Messenger on computers, laptops, and tablets. Using these platforms required some technological knowledge, and for that the younger siblings who still lived with their parents were essential.

During one home visit, I observed Thomas, the younger brother of Leela who worked as a nurse in Canada, providing such technical support to their mother Anna. As soon as I found my spot on the sofa, Anna brought a small laptop from another room, sat next to me, and opened the device on her lap. She tried to connect to Facebook to show me some photos, but something "didn't work properly." She could open the internet browser but then could not continue to Facebook. After several attempts, she complained to Thomas, and he disappeared into another room to check the internet connection. He had installed a Wi-Fi connection at the house only a few months earlier. Usually they would have the laptop, together with two small speakers, placed on a desk in one of the two bedrooms, but this time they brought the laptop out to the sitting area for me to see. After Thomas fixed the connection, Anna managed to open her Facebook profile, adding with a laugh that she normally knew how to open things unless "Thomas does something" to the system. She showed me the photos of Leela, her husband, and their toddler son, and the photos of herself visiting the young family when they had lived in Singapore. "The further away she moves, the closer our relationship becomes," noted Anna with a smile.

Around 7:00 P.M., Leela's father, then mother, then Thomas each called her on the phone multiple times, but Leela did not answer. It was still early where she lived, about 8:00 A.M. To deal with the time difference between Kerala and Canada, Anna explained that she usually stayed up late in the night to talk to Leela at a time that suited her daughter better, which was midmorning. Although the family referred to their video calls as "Skype," it appeared that they did not use that platform at all. Thomas mentioned that he had never even downloaded Skype because it took up too much disk space on the laptop; they only used Facebook Messenger. At last, a ringing sound came from the laptop, and a sleepy Leela, wearing a yellow sweater with her hair tied in a bun, waved at us, smiling. Soon, her husband and 2-year-old son joined her. We passed the laptop around so she could see me, and we exchanged a few introductory remarks.

When the laptop landed back in Anna's lap, Leela left to take a shower, and Anna started playing with her grandson who remained seated in front of the screen by himself. Suddenly, something went wrong with the sound: the microphone and speakers integrated into the laptop went silent. Immediately afterward, Leela's husband called on the landline, and Anna started entertaining her grandson by making baby sounds on the phone. Meanwhile, Thomas fetched a set of external speakers from his room, attached them to the laptop, and told Anna that she could speak without the phone. It was fascinating to observe how deeply Anna became immersed in the interaction with her grandson via webcam, to the point of not noticing the humdrum of visitors and the failing technology.

Since digital technologies demanded specific skills and technological knowledge, they impacted on gender and seniority-based hierarchies within families by increasing the reliance of the parents on their youngest children. Commonly, the head of the household was the father, but digital technologies could change that to a certain degree. In her family, Mary had the essential technological skills that were needed to establish a webcam connection between her household and the two sisters in the United Kingdom. I observed this in person when Mary and her parents invited me to stay with them for a few days. One evening, Mary called her middle sister Susy and her husband, whom Mary called by his kinship term *Achacha* ("Brother"), on Skype through the family laptop. Nobody answered, so she tried calling her oldest sister instead. No reply either. On a second try, *Achacha* picked up Mary's call via Skype on his smartphone. Mary then positioned the external webcam so that he could see both me, sitting at the desk, and her, sitting on the bed. A few minutes later, Mary's mother and father joined us in the room and Mary stood up to give them space on the bed: her mother in the center, looking directly at the webcam, and her father beside her.

The laptop, provided by Susy, was intended for the whole family's use, so Mary, her mother, and her father had equal access to it, at least physically. However, the device—hardware and software combined—required certain knowledge and skills that only Mary possessed. Her father, by contrast, did not have the necessary skills and therefore had little power to create and maintain the webcam interaction. When this particular call was over, he quietly retreated into the living room to watch TV. In this way, the laptop gave Mary considerable control over this field event and over other daily webcam interactions with her sisters abroad (see chapter 2; Ahlin and Li 2019). The technological expertise required to create transnational care collectives thus superseded the family hierarchies of gender, age, and individual ownership of the device.

Further, image-based digital technologies contributed to extending the collectives beyond kin and helped to strengthen non-kin relations that would otherwise remain weaker. For Sonia and Ajay, whose son John worked in Guyana while their daughter was studying nursing in another Indian state, the transnational care collective involved a shopkeeper and his tiny shop by the main road, where he sold anything from colorful candy and cigarettes to pens and peanuts. Ajay regularly went there to buy mobile phone credit, and he only had to walk for about fifteen minutes on the dirt road winding through the rubber trees to reach the shop. The shopkeeper topped Ajay's phone with credit, and during one of Ajay's first visits the shopkeeper also instructed the old man on how to check the credit balance on his phone. The shopkeeper's contribution could be seen as minor, but it was a key part to maintaining the transnational care collective because their interaction enabled Ajay to take care of his digital device and thus maintain his relationship with his son abroad.

Digital technologies additionally deepened the relationship between nurses' parents who lived alone and their "good friends" who lived close to the parents in Kerala. Significantly, I only noticed this kind of non-kin relationship in families where the nurse abroad was male. One mother told me, "Our son recently moved to Australia and has given us the numbers of his friends who are very helpful. He told us to call his friends in time of need." After a male nurse's departure abroad, his friends could become quite involved in the life of his parents, to the point of becoming "family friends."

I noticed how close these young men sometimes were to the parents through the fact that they would join the interview sessions, if only to be silently present. In one family, for example, I was welcomed by the two parents, by their daughter who lived in Kerala and was visiting for a few days, and by Anand, a man in his 40s who owned a shop next to the parents' house. Anand was the one who stood by the road waiting for me and my driver to point us to the right driveway. The father described Anand as a "very good friend" of their son who lived in the UAE. Their son reportedly called regularly and was about to visit them soon. Anand sometimes helped the older couple by calling their son on Skype via his smartphone. For that purpose, the father would walk to Anand's shop nearby where the internet connection was better, although the mother could not join him because of her injured knee.

The good friends of sons were therefore engaged to occasionally visit the parents to check on them in person as well as to establish a webcam connection between the migrating sons and their parents. By recruiting their friends into their transnational care collective, migrating sons made sure that their parents were doing well, particularly in relation to health—they realized that their parents might not easily share health problems with them (see chapter 6).

Digital technologies thus intensified the non-kin relationship between parents and sons' good friends. This relationship, however, was not always possible or easily available. Sonia and Ajay's son John, for example, noted that—for some reason unknown to me—he did not have many social connections in his own village and thus was not able to ask any friends for help. Other male nurses admitted that such care connections were not entirely based on selfless friendship but were at least partially stimulated by money. Aaron, who was an only son and lived in the United Kingdom, mentioned that he paid 20 or 30 British pounds (USD 25–30) every once in a while to his friends who helped his parents. This kind of support was vital for Aaron's father who had chronic obstructive pulmonary disease (COPD) and required regular oxygen tanks replacements (see chapter 6). "I give them some money for their time and effort, so they're happy," Aaron told me on a WhatsApp video call, catching his breath while he climbed a city street in the United Kingdom on his way to a shopping mall.

Yet another non-kin involved in the transnational care collectives were healthcare professionals at the nurses' workplaces, particularly specialist doctors. Several nurses, including Sara (see chapter 1), told me that they refrained from discussing their parents' health issues with their doctors in Kerala in order not to disrespect local professional hierarchies and thereby endanger the relationship between their parents and their doctor. By contrast, the nurses were more open toward discussing their parents' health—and the health issues of extended family members—with the doctors in their own workplace. When I visited her in Muscat, Oman, Usha recounted,

If anybody in my family in Kerala needs medical advice, I ask the doctors here in my hospital for it. See, this hospital is not like in Muscat—these doctors here are all nice. They are Egyptians, Pakistani, Bangladeshi, they come from many countries. They know us nurses personally, they are not calling me "Sister," they call me by name, so close we are. Yesterday my mother told me that her sister had a problem, some swelling or a cyst in her breast. When I was on duty, I asked one of the doctors here for advice. He told me what to ask her—was it possible to move the swelling or not? How big was it? And some other questions. I told my mother on the phone what his questions were, and she asked her sister. So my mother got all the answers, and I discussed them with the doctor again. He said that if it's movable, then it's no problem. If it's not movable, it's dangerous. Then the doctor said that she could go to the hospital and ask for a biopsy. Yesterday she went to the hospital, they did the biopsy, but they haven't got the results yet.

Similarly, Teena, who worked in the Maldives, told me on the phone that she was on friendly terms with the doctors in her hospital. There were thirty-five nurses from India, and many of the doctors were their compatriots, mainly from northern India. Because of the age difference—the doctors were generally in their 40s or 50s while nurses were in their 20s and early 30s—Teena said that the doctors treated the nurses "as their children":

> They are like family, [and] we can talk to them about anything. Once, when my mother had a heart problem, I even put her cardiologist in India on the phone with the cardiologist in my hospital. They discussed the condition, what medicines were needed and so on. Together, they helped to determine how serious the condition was and whether it was important for me to return home. In this case, I indeed returned home for a visit. It's just an hour's flight, and the ticket costs less than US $100.

Digital technologies are thus at the intersection of multiple relations that only begin with those of aging parents and their migrating children. The devices help establish social relations outside this dyad, whether virtually or face to face, with other family members such as the nurses' younger siblings or their own children, as well as with non-kin, from shopkeepers to nurses' friends and doctors outside India. Transnational care collectives are therefore not stable entities, nor are they limited to the closest family members. Quite the contrary, the collectives allow, and sometimes require, different kinds and levels of connection within and beyond the parent–child relationship. Which relationships are needed for transnational care collectives to function through time is a matter of circumstance, including the changing technological skills, abilities, and health conditions of the people concerned.

CALLING AS A CARE PRACTICE

One afternoon, a hired driver took me and Elisa, my assistant, to a village outside Kottayam for a home visit. The settlement was overlooked by a church on a small hill. The left side of the slope was crowded with small single-story houses with limited driveway space, mostly without gates, and with barely any garden land around them. Still, many had been renovated, and I could almost smell the fresh paint of their tiffany blue, mint green, and carnation pink façades. Here lived Sonia and Ajay. They welcomed us into their home, and during our conversation I inquired about how they communicated with John.

"We have a landline phone," Sonia explained. "So we just have to attend to it when he calls us here. We don't know how to handle the mobile phone. If we get a call on the mobile, I can identify the number before I take the call. The children showed me how to take and cancel a call. That is all that I know."

Among the families I encountered it was common for the children to call their parents rather than the opposite. The children felt more skilled in calling, especially when this involved VoIP and the use of devices and software programs other than simple phones. As Sonia mentioned, she did not feel comfortable

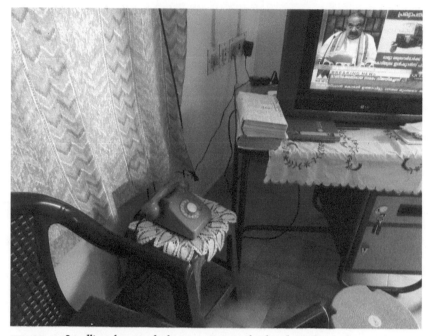

FIGURE 4.3. Landline phone and television, commonly placed together in the room corner.

making mobile calls and was not even sure which number she should call to reach John. Some parents noted that their children's "duty," or work obligations, was a priority, and they did not want to disturb them. Additionally, by being the first to call, their children automatically assumed the costs, which was yet another way of providing financial care. The cases when parents initiated communication were exceptional and related to circumstances that had a sense of urgency.

In the same village, just a short walk away, lived another couple with children abroad. Upon hearing our voices in front of the gate, Sosha emerged from the house in a brown hued, worn-out sari. She was home alone while her husband was away for work in another town. The main door of the house opened directly into a living room, and my eyes and ears were immediately drawn to the small, old TV in the corner, and a landline phone sitting right next to it (figure 4.3). The TV was on, but the image and sound were not clear.

Sosha had been peeling jackfruit, the skin coming off on the newspaper sheets spread across the floor in the middle of the living room. There, she sat us down and served us juice, then jackfruit fried in coconut oil; bright yellow kernels glittered like a thousand little suns on a white plate. It was a jackfruit season, and Sosha had plucked plenty of this produce from her garden, stocking her freezer especially for one of her daughters who loved it most.

Sosha had three daughters, all nurses. One worked in the United Kingdom, another in South Africa, and the third in UAE. When I asked her about how she kept in touch them, Sosha's face brightened up instantly. She talked to them daily, up to one hour with each of them, and their conversations were scheduled from around 8:00 P.M. to 10:00 P.M., based on different time zones and her daughters' work schedules. Sosha only used her landline phone for this purpose (before her youngest daughter had emigrated, they also used to talk on Skype). For Sosha, these daily conversations were a lifesaver: without them, she would worry herself sick about her daughters. "If they don't call on time, I give them a missed call. If they still don't call back, I can't sleep the whole night!"

The practice of calling as a form of care at a distance became particularly evident when it was not delivered: the parents perceived a lack of calls as a signal for concern. Among all the families I met, in two of them their relationships had been so poor before migration that the family members had no contact over digital technologies after their adult children migrated abroad (see Manju's story in chapter 3). In other families, however, failure to call on the part of the children alarmed their parents and made them anxious, triggering worry about the well-being of their children and about how the physical distance would impact their relationship.

To appease their worries, the parents would go to great lengths to reach their child abroad. Standing in her garden, where her son's good friend was hunting for the best Wi-Fi connection to make a video call (figure 4.4), Viju's mother told me,

> When Viju left for the U.K. for the very first time, it took about two weeks for him to call us. He had never stayed away from us. He was in a place he had no idea about. In between, there was a family whom we knew and who also had some family members in the U.K. We called them, and they contacted one of their relatives in the U.K., and later Viju called us. We were really destroyed. Viju also didn't know how we felt. It was like he had left us for good.

Without any contact, Viju's mother felt as though their relationship had been abruptly broken, invoking in her feelings of intense concern, abandonment, and even grief. The absence of any phone calls could mean that something unfortunate had happened to their son. After Viju's parents had invested so much effort into tracking him down through acquaintances, he realized how important it was for him to call home because this mattered to his parents greatly. He was not used to calling them regularly when he studied in another Indian state, but after he had migrated internationally he came to see calling as a necessary way to communicate to his parents that he was doing well and, furthermore, that he still cared about and for them. As Viju told me with a serious look on his face, he subsequently made sure to call them regularly.

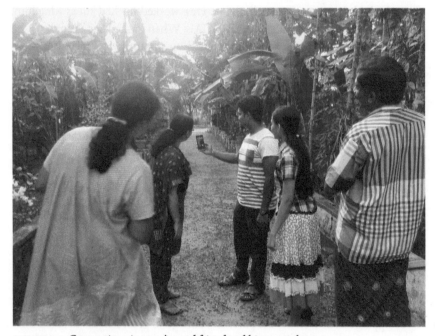

FIGURE 4.4. Connecting via a son's good friend and his smartphone.

In transnational families, children had to find new ways to compensate for the impossibility of being physically together, to dispel their parents' worries about them as well as to mitigate their feelings of abandonment. At a distance, children could give their attention most effectively via digital technologies, particularly through phone calls. Anthony explicitly related his regular calling home to care:

> I think care is the understanding and trust; it's not touching, it's not giving money, it's the feeling that you have—it's love. But there are different ways to express it. Some people never express it. Some people are overexpressive even without having that much care in their mind. Well, I call my parents all the time, but I don't tell them, "Mommy, I love you; Daddy, I love you," but I *call* [emphasis] them every day. That's a gesture. That's how I show my love. I call them every day, I speak to them, [and] I'm well informed; and they discuss everything with me, [and] I discuss everything with them.

Remittances are important in reconceptualizing international migration as a care practice (chapter 5), but Anthony pointed out that money is not the central actor in enacting care at a distance. Rather, in transnational care collectives the most significant practice of care is the act of *calling*. This practice is dependent on strong affective relationships, which could be linked to a range of emotions, from love to feelings of duty, indebtedness, and even guilt. Indeed, affect emerged as the main stimulus that keeps the transnational care collectives going.

As one young female nurse told me, "Even if you are sitting nearby but don't feel for your parents, that doesn't help. It's about having a feeling for your parents from the heart, a genuine feeling. We should be near—I know the importance of that. But they should feel that I care for them, [and] there's a mutual understanding. That's a good relationship, [and] it won't go away even in many years." In this way, affect transpired as a significant impetus for migrating children to pick up their phone and call their parents' number again and again, every day.

FREQUENT CALLING AS GOOD CARE

If calling through digital technologies is a new way of enacting care at a distance, how to establish when such care is good? With little previous guidance on the norms of technologically mediated care, family members tinkered with the frequency of calling to determine through negotiation what good care at a distance could be. When I asked family members about how they kept in touch with each other, I often received the same response: daily. Most nurses, like Sara and Benny, called their parents once or several times a day, while others, like John, called once to several times a week. Anthony, for instance, said, "I speak to my parents every day on the phone. I ring them, and we talk for ten to fifteen minutes or even more than that." For calling to be considered good care, then, it is not sufficient to do it sometimes—calling has to be done frequently. How frequent is frequent enough depends on each transnational care collective and its members.

Frequency of calling was further entwined with regularity. Rather than calling spontaneously, the children and their parents tinkered with calling times to accommodate different time zones, work schedules, and pastime activities. In this way, they established when would be best to call, and eventually they began to adhere to those particular times of the day. For example, when discussing their calling habits, Sosha pointed to the clock above the TV set and said she waited for each of her daughters to call at a particular hour, which correlated well with the time zones and work schedules of her daughters' various locations.

Similarly, when calling home, Sara considered both her work and her family members' personal habits. She finished her morning duty at 3:00 P.M., returned home, had a bite for lunch, and slept for an hour. She usually started work early in the morning, so her family let her rest in the afternoon. Then she called her daughter at 5:15 P.M. Indian time. Sara knew that from 6:00 to 8:00 P.M. her mother watched television, around 8:00 to 9:00 P.M. her parents would pray, and from 9:00 to 10:00 P.M. they watched another television serial. Sara called her parents after prayer, at about 8:30 P.M. their time, taking into account the 1.5-hour time difference. Sara's husband watched television with his mother, then they cooked and finished their dinner at about 11:00 P.M., which was 9:30 P.M. in Oman. That's when Sara usually called him.

Paying attention to time in this way gave Sara's calls a certain structure, and it transformed this everyday interaction into a routine. After a period of tinkering, these relations mediated through digital technologies eventually became regularized and systematized to accommodate schedules of all those involved. Phoning outside these routine times indicated that some problem or emergency had occurred. To avoid confusion and worry, Sara always informed her parents in advance if she knew that she would be unable to call them at the expected hour:

> If I'm busy at work, I can't call, so they know that I'm on duty. I tell them in advance. [If] I don't call for two or three days, even if it is because of my work schedule, then my father would say, "Ha, are you also becoming like your brothers? Have you changed your mind, you are only calling us weekly now?" He will ask like that, and then I will know he is feeling . . . sad that I'm not calling. That's why he's jokingly complaining.[3]

That frequent calling had become a new norm of good care was most clearly visible when this norm was breached, and complete lack of contact through digital technologies was considered a new form of abandonment. That was the case for Manju (see chapter 3) whose daughter was a nurse in a Gulf country. Manju was deeply saddened that her daughter was not in touch with her in any way, and she complained that "she never calls." In India, letting one's parents live in a shelter is considered neglectful on the part of the children, but for Manju the abandonment was exacerbated by the lack of phone calls from her daughter. Not calling at all, or not doing so frequently enough, came to be interpreted as poor care, and could even be considered a new way of "doing neglect" and abandonment at a distance.

COLLECTIVE CARE

At the beginning of my research, I set out to study eldercare, but through my fieldwork I found that it is almost impossible to look at transnational eldercare exclusively. Scholars of transnationalism have suggested that in transnational families care "circulates" such that the focus of care shifts from one family member to another, depending on who is in most need of it at a given moment (Baldassar and Merla 2014). When looking at care as practice, however, it becomes difficult to talk about its direction because a single practice can be meaningful as care for more than one actor involved in the care collective, albeit in different ways. In this context, care is then rarely just eldercare but is rather intergenerational family care.

Following the proposition that in a care collective the object of care is not one single person but the collective itself (see chapter 1; Winance 2010), I argue that the object of care in transnational families is not the aging parents but the digitally connected families. This formulation highlights that in transnational care collectives the care is shared and distributed among the parents, their children and others (especially grandchildren), and even the digital technologies.

Children as the Object of Care

As I observed Ashu, fully engrossed in her smartphone, I realized that for her daily calling was more than just a new duty of eldercare. At least for some nurses, calling home was also a practice of self-care. Through frequent calling, digital technologies mitigated the feelings of abandonment on the side of the parents, but they also alleviated the feelings of loneliness and homesickness of the migrated adult children. This was especially the case for female nurses who were abroad alone. The three nurses I stayed with in Oman—Sara, Margaret, and Ashu—preferred to live alone rather than sharing a residence with their work colleagues, and at the same time they put considerable effort into maintaining social contact with their family members and friends through digital media.

"I'm not the only one calling my parents. My brothers are doing that too, but not every day; it's not possible for them," Sara stated, as she started explaining to me her many daily calls from Oman to her family in Kerala:

> Maybe one brother calls every fifteen days, [and] the other one is sending text messages in between his calls. Because they are all busy with their own families. Like in every family, maybe the husband is going to work, the wife has to look after their children; then the wife is going to work, and the husband has to look after the children. So I must understand their situation. But I'm free, no? After duty, I have no other obligations, [so] I'm free, and I can call. That's why my parents know I am always calling. What else is there for me to do?

Sara laughed at her rhetorical question. In explaining the difference between how often her brothers and she called their parents, she emphasized her availability and lack of obligations next to work.

But Sara's freedom also entailed and emerged from being alone. Her lifestyle in Oman was a great contrast to the common way of living in Kerala where a woman like her, middle-aged and married with children, would be embedded in a broad family network and involved in one social event after another. For Sara, living alone in Oman was a personal choice, but it was also related to age and finances. The women who opted to stay by themselves were in their 40s or older, meaning that their children were already teenagers or young adults. Husbands had sometimes tried to join them, but often they struggled with finding employment in Oman, and so their presence was deemed more valuable in Kerala (chapter 5). There, at least they could help their aging parents and in-laws. By contrast, nurses of childbearing years preferred to have their husbands living with them, even if they were unemployed, so they could help with raising small children. Additionally, some husbands, especially in families who lived in Muscat, did manage to find well-paying jobs in branches such as travel, marketing, and sales.

In some other Gulf countries, however, young nurses had little choice but to live without their close family in dormitories shared with other colleagues who came from all over Asia. For them, digital technologies were a vital connection to their family in Kerala, which sustained their emotional and mental well-being. Among these nurses was Joy, a young, unmarried woman who was spending her second year working in Saudi Arabia. In our conversation, Joy noted that it was difficult for her to move around outside the immediate environment of the hospital and the dormitory because she did not wear the black cloak called an abaya or the head cover, hijab, as expected of women in Saudi Arabia. The obvious markers of her identity—her dress as well as the tone of her skin, the little jewelry she wore, and her visible hair—indicated that she was a foreign, South Asian, Christian woman, and this differentiation made her feel uncomfortable and unsafe outside the hospital where she worked and the hostel where she stayed. This was not only Joy's experience; in previous research, nurses living in Saudi Arabia had reported that they had a hard time due to the substantial differences between the local population and migrating workers, including nationality-based discrimination at work (Alshareef et al. 2020; Osella and Osella 2008; Percot 2006).

One tactic that helped Joy cope with the harsh conditions of her life abroad was keeping in touch with her mother daily through the landline phone, mobile phone, and Skype interchangeably. Among these options, Joy favored Skype. Talking through the webcam, she said, had a "good impact on [her] well-being" when she was missing her home and was finding it challenging to be so far away. She felt much better, she said, every time her mother made a dish and showed it to her through the screen. I asked her if it did not make her sad not to be able to share the meal with her family, to touch, taste, and smell it. Without hesitation Joy replied, "No, it makes me feel soooo happy! Just to see, it's enough!"

Beyond offering emotional support, parents cared for their children in relation to their physical health, especially in critical situations like giving birth. In Kerala, I observed one mother offer postpartum advice through Skype to her daughter, a nurse who had just given birth in the United Kingdom. After instructing her to stay indoors for a certain amount of time, the mother went on to explain how to use some Ayurvedic remedies that she had sent to the United Kingdom through a common acquaintance. In yet another family, the parents intervened from a distance when their daughter abroad was suffering from domestic violence. One day the mother received a call from her son-in-law only to realize that he was being aggressive toward her daughter while on the phone. With a friend's assistance, the parents called the police in the United Kingdom and requested an intervention. To their great relief, their son-in-law was arrested within half an hour. The phone thus emerged as an invaluable device that helped to save their daughter's life and possibly that of their grandchild.

Despite people's hopes and best intentions, mobility does not necessarily improve the lives of migrants, nor does it automatically contribute to harmonious family relationships; on the contrary, migration may have quite the opposite effect (Gallo 2006; George 2005; Percot 2012; see also Gamburd 2000). Difficult transitions and troubled relationships, whether marital or professional, are not always easy to share with family at home. However, the webcam is good at revealing even that which people would prefer to keep secret. Joy's mother, for example, explained to me that by regularly seeing her daughter on Skype she could continuously monitor Joy's health and well-being beyond what her daughter shared with her on the phone. Through the webcam, she closely inspected Joy's physical appearance: "Does she look thin? Does she look pale? Is she eating enough? Is she smiling enough? Or is her face sad and worried?" By tracing subtle changes of her face and gestures, Joy's mother was looking for clues of concealed unhappiness and strain. This allowed her to notice any trouble quickly and immediately offer emotional support and encouragement.

Through the webcam, the observer may feel that they are "perceiving 'more truth'" and "having a better access to reality compared to words, and hence, to the telephone" (Pols 2011, 460). On the other hand, those being observed are well aware of the power of the webcam to reveal too much and potentially show what they would prefer not to share. In the case of migrating children, this could be anything from feelings of sadness to poor living conditions. "I wouldn't want my mother to see that; it would only make her sad and worried," one nurse who planned to migrate soon after our meeting told me. "If I didn't have a nice room, I would just say that the webcam is not working"—he laughed as he strategized his way out of unpleasant webcam revelations. I write further about secrecy in transnational care collectives in chapter 6, where I describe how parents, too, avoided revealing certain information, especially related to ill health.

Caring for Digital Technologies

A compelling insight about care collectives is that the object of care is dispersed among its heterogenous members, humans and technologies alike (chapter 1; Winance 2010). As my fieldwork showed, digital technologies not only enable parents and their children to provide care to each other, but they also demand care for themselves.

To start with, prepaid mobile phones had to be constantly topped up with credit. This could be done easily at any small shop where the shopkeeper had the appropriate license. Such shops were common even outside towns and were

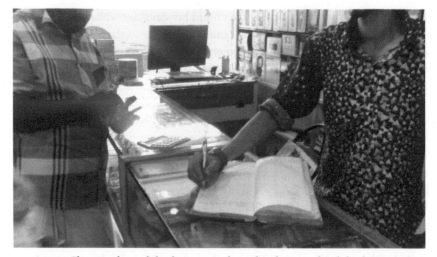

FIGURE 4.5. Charging the mobile phone; note the wide selection of mobile phones in the background.

usually situated only a short stroll from almost any house. Many older adults mentioned that they recharged their mobile phones themselves, although women often asked their husbands to do it for them. In one local shop, I noticed that the process of credit recharging was quick and uncomplicated. The shopkeeper recorded in a notebook the phone number to be recharged and the amount that the customer, most of whom were men, wished to upload; this was usually about INR 50–60, or less than USD 1 (figure 4.5). After receiving the payment, the shopkeeper processed the request through his own mobile phone, and the customers received a text message confirming a successful recharge.

What happened if digital technologies were not properly taken care of? Sitting in the closed veranda, surrounded by tall, lean rubber trees, Sonia and Ajay told me about the trouble they had experienced when they neglected their landline and mobile phone. "We can't call on the mobile when the balance is over," Ajay started. "At least the landline doesn't stop working in the middle of the conversation."

"With the landline, even if we fail to pay the bill on time, we can call," Sonia continued. "With the mobile, if there is no balance, no matter how much we try to call we can't. I surely get angry if the connection breaks! Just as we are about to know about each other's well-being, the balance in the mobile is over, and the connection cut abruptly. Wouldn't anyone get angry?"

So different kinds of technologies not only support care practices, but they also demand specific kinds of care. This care is primarily about paying attention to their operational needs: mobile phones must be charged with credit and energy, landline phones must have all their lines in order, and in both cases the telecommunication service must be paid and properly connected. The practical care for technologies was provided by the children, who sent money and sometimes digital devices from abroad, and by the parents, who paid the bills, plugged in the battery charger, contacted the phone company for repairs, and avoided breakage or other damage to the equipment.

The attention paid to technologies may be motivated by various affective values, such as friendship or fun (Pols and Moser 2009). But Sonia's comment about becoming angry when the devices stopped functioning indicates that her own motivation to take care of digital technologies was fueled by values of strong kin relations. Through caring for their technologies, family members took care of their relationships.

MUNDANE MATTERS

At the same time as they contribute to enacting care at a distance, digital technologies shape, in subtle ways, how family members relate to each other through the kind of content that can be shared through them. The materiality of digital devices is significant here because different devices afford the users to engage with them in various ways (Fisher 2004; Costa 2018). Migration and media scholars have argued that in transnational families the gesture of calling is key for family relations, and the act is even more important than the content of the daily conversations, which revolve around "insignificant" details of everyday life (Licoppe 2004; Licoppe and Smoreda 2005; Wilding 2006). But why would people talk about seemingly trivial, meaningless, and prosaic things every day, sometimes for hours?

"Sharing Everydayness" on the Phone

In the families that I met, the content of daily phone conversations generally revolved around the mundane details of day-to-day life. Ashu, for example, told me that she always first asked her mother how she was and if she needed anything, specifically any medicine for her problem with hypertension. Ashu then inquired about the animals her mother had—the goat, one dog, and two cats— and then about the neighbors' children and other people living nearby and the church. In this way, she was always "well informed" about what was happening with her mother and her wider home community. Beyond monitoring health, Ashu's aim behind frequent calling was not to inquire about something specific or to exchange a particular piece of information but to participate in her mother's life through inquiring about the mundane details of her days.

Such comprehensive phone accounts of everyday life could also become a source of tension, leading to situations that were uncomfortable for the conversation partners. Mathew, a young nurse working in Australia, increased the number of calls home significantly after migrating abroad. When he had lived in another Indian state during his studies, he "only called his parents when he had to ask them for money," as Mathew's friend who joined our meeting half-jokingly said. Moving within the country for studies was a sort of preparation for migrating internationally but with important differences.

Despite the immense geographic distances within India, the children could return home more easily than from abroad. They were still Indian nationals, so they felt quite at home, and as students they had not yet assumed the responsibilities of providing care for their parents. However, once they were abroad, their status changed: they became "migrants" and "foreigners," and they were potentially subject to racial, ethnic, religious, and sexual discrimination that they might have not experienced in their own country. Their flight across one or the other ocean also shifted their position within their family from being a dependent child to an adult child who should be able to—and ought to—send home remittances and thereby become a carer. Returning home was neither as affordable nor as easy to arrange as hopping on a train that would take them from any part of India to Kerala within a matter of hours.

For Matthew, the increased frequency of calling home was in a way a self-care practice, too. But because of the intensification of contact after his migration, Mathew and his mother ran into problems concerning what to discuss. As Mathew's mother said,

> Of course, we are sad about Mathew being in Australia. But since he calls us every day, we don't miss him that much. He informs us of everything. He keeps telling us, "Say something, say . . . What news is there?" What is there to talk so much every day? We say the same thing again and again. We usually talk between fifteen and twenty minutes. What is there to talk about every day? Because he calls every day. So he asks about the plants, the domestic animals, neighbors, and so on.

Mathew's mother made a weary face, indicating that she sometimes struggled with their phone interaction. When she had exhausted the repertoire of news that she deemed important to share, she was not sure what more to say. And yet she did not attenuate the conversation but instead resorted to talking about domestic animals and plants, filling the time with what could be considered mundane or banal small talk.

In this way, both Mathew and his mother adjusted to the new context in which their relationship was taking place, across two continents connected by digital technologies. For Mathew's mother, the calls, and her persistence with them, were a way to take care of Mathew and reduce his homesickness, ensuring that he remained part of the domestic realm. Again, this highlights that care within the transnational care collectives was not unidirectional but dispersed among its members.

Although the content of these interactions may seem inconsequential at first glance, the daily exchange of details on the phone enabled transnational family members to create and maintain a kind of "shared everydayness" at a distance.

This demanded quite some work: tinkering to find the most appropriate time and type of digital technologies, caring for these technologies, maintaining the regularity of calling, and finding ways to keep the conversation going. The labor involved in this practice shows that "sharing everydayness" at a distance did not happen by itself—people had to work together with the technologies to actively construct it.

Yet despite the substantial effort that went into frequently calling home, none of the nurses I talked to complained, even indirectly, about calling their parents daily as any sort of financial, practical, or emotional burden. Clearly, frequent calling has become a new filial duty, and duties are to be fulfilled; complaining about them is simply senseless (Bomhoff 2011, 131–132).

"Spending Time Together" through a Webcam

Being together face-to-face involves not only speaking but sometimes also being silent. On the phone, silence as a type of nonverbal communication may be problematic, given that this technology is designed specifically for verbal communication. As Ann Goelitz (2003) found in her study of telephone support for family caregivers, silence on the phone can be hard because it is impossible to see what the other person is doing. Silence is difficult to interpret: something might be wrong with the technological connection, or with the relation between the conversation partners, or information might intentionally be withheld. To overcome this issue, Mathew and his mother turned their conversation into detailed descriptions of daily life, a strategy used not only to share "what news is there" but also to fill the silences and to be together apart.

If silence as an ingredient of being together is problematic on the phone because people cannot see each other, what happens when image is added to sound, as is the case with the webcam? I found that the effect of the image is transformed through frequency in a paradoxical way. The materiality of the webcam allows its users to relate to each other differently than via the phone. With daily use of the webcam, the significance of image as something that is meaningful because it is visible fades away as the family members concentrate on being together without words and even without looking at each other.

When visiting Mary's home in Kerala, I noted the following experience of webcam interaction. It took place just after Mary's sister, Susy, who was pregnant, finished her checkup in the hospital and was driving home with her husband and their toddler son.

From U.K., Susy calls home to Kerala through Skype on her mobile phone. At first she's pointing the phone to her face so that we're looking at her directly, but the picture is very blurry, and she doesn't seem to be very interested in our picture. She's not very talkative, she appears tired or maybe concerned. She is holding the phone on her lefthand side, below; perhaps she has placed it on her knee. She's not looking at her phone, into the webcam, but we see her face from below as her eyes are fixed on the road. She says that all was well in the hospital. After that, we ride with them, through the camera, in silence. The following several moments seem quite magical—it's as if we are all sitting in the same car, looking out the same grey sky somewhere (where?) above London. The conversation is not taking place all the time, just as if we were all in the same car. There's no real focus, nothing much to do, we're just all taking the drive back home.

While Susy and her family were sitting in their car, on the other end of the webcam Mary and I sat in the chairs at the table while her parents sat on the bed. After exchanging the most important piece of information about Susy's checkup we were all quiet for most of the time, staring at the laptop in front of us. No specific information was exchanged; we were all just "traveling together" for a while. This interaction, full of interruptions and silences, lasted for about ten minutes.

In contrast to the phone, silence on the webcam is not problematic because it does not signal a break in communication—at any moment, everyone can see what is happening on the other side of the screen. But the webcam does more than just allow for silence. Paradoxically, because it affords seeing other people, it is not necessary anymore to look at the webcam continuously. In this way, the webcam enables "spending time together" at a distance, which is a different way to relate to each other than through "sharing everydayness" on the phone.

The way transnational families spent time together on the webcam is distinct from a Skype interaction set up as a meeting with the goal to talk about a specific topic. In professional settings, including in health care, the conversation partners tend to sit in front of their computers and gaze at the screen, careful not to move out of the webcam frame (Pols 2012, 102). Using the webcam in this way creates a meeting-like experience, with the specific purpose of sharing certain information. By contrast, Mary's family members called each other on the webcam every day and did not follow any sort of formality characteristic of Skype meetings in which the date, time, and topic are predetermined. Frequency was not the only factor in fostering spending time together on webcam. Familiarity between family members was important, too; the relationship between parents and children, underpinned by personal affect and attachment, is not the same as professional relationships.

Through a material semiotic analysis of frequent calling, I have argued that care is a relational process that includes not only people but also nonhuman entities such as everyday digital technologies. When family members are scattered across the world, care practices that demand physical proximity, although still considered important, become impossible to follow. In this situation, parents and their children tinker with digital technologies to discover how these devices can help them establish new forms of care that can indeed be practiced across vast geographic distances. Together, the adult children, aging parents, and technologies form transnational care collectives in which people adjust, tinker, and negotiate what care at a distance could be and how it should be done to be considered good. In this context, the emphasis moves from practices that require being together physically—such as sharing a residence and food—to practices that include digital technologies such as frequent calling, sharing everydayness on the phone, and spending time together on the webcam.

Expressions like "keeping in touch" and "staying in contact" (Baldassar 2008; Baldassar, Nedelcu, and Wilding 2016) emphasize the importance of the gesture of calling for family relationships to continue across continents. Similarly, science and technology studies scholar Judy Wajcman (2016, 149) noted that "the call or text itself may be constitutive of the relationship." In the families that I met, daily calling meant "I call, and through this I do care." In this way, people expressed their feelings of love and trust, but also their worries, loneliness, and fear of being abandoned. Care became enacted through everyday actions such as making calls, taking calls, coordinating time zones, being silent together, and talking about or showing faces, food, and ferns on the webcam. People built on such practices to connect and maintain caring relations at a distance while simultaneously embedded in their various physical environments. At the same time, care became distributed among all members of the collective because the object of care was not only the aging parents but also the children and even the digital technologies. In line with Winance's observation (2010), care was collective, and, simultaneously, the collective was cared for.

Finally, sharing everydayness on the phone and spending time together on the webcam emerged as two practices that highlight what kind of care people are trying to achieve through frequent contact via digital technologies. The notion of sharing everydayness on the phone considers conversations about everyday details as far from trivial; rather, talking about the weather, domestic plants, animals, neighbors, their children, and the church congregations was significant precisely because these things were ordinary—people organized their lives around them. Actively constructing everydayness by sharing detailed accounts of the quotidian via digital technologies thus enabled people to enact everydayness and share a life even when sharing a residence was not an option.

5 · SHIFTING DUTIES

As my fieldwork advanced and the more attention I paid to people's experiences of migration, the more evident it became that digital technologies are not the only nonhuman actor that make transnational care collectives possible. A new actor emerged: money, appearing in several shapes such as educational fees, loans, and remittances. Money, it became clear, is significantly involved in the project and process of international migration, and as such it is crucial for the creation of transnational care collectives. After all, an essential feature of these collectives is their transnational character.

National and international migration both introduce geographic distance among family members, but they do so in different ways. Matthew, for example, had almost never called home when he was studying nursing in another Indian state, but the frequency of his calls to his parents increased drastically once he moved to Australia for work (chapter 4). In this chapter, I explore how money contributes to the making and shaping of transnational care collectives through the investigation of filial duties, especially those of daughters. Such a focus brings to light new layers of complexity in gender and kinship dynamics in transnational families beyond the husband–wife relationship, which scholarly work has previously addressed (e.g., Bhalla 2008; Gallo 2005; George 2005; Percot 2012). As I showed in chapter 3, in the discourse of abandonment migrating children are criticized for leaving their parents behind and thereby neglecting the basic filial duties that are only possible through physical co-presence. But how do these adult children see themselves, and how are they perceived by their own parents?

To address this question, I draw on empirical ethics (Pols 2013), an approach that is fruitful to understand how a nonhuman actor such as money can contribute to reshaping what it means to be a good child—and particularly a good daughter—in a transnational setting. Empirical ethics help to understand how the good in care is achieved through everyday tinkering, exploring, and modifying within social, material, and, I would add, affective relations (see chapter 1). What is considered good, then, is not simply a matter of judging how well people align themselves according to some external ideals or norms; it is "something to do, in practice, as care goes on" (Mol, Moser, and Pols 2010, 13). As a "practical achievement" (Winance 2007), good care is locally situated, based on constant work, and subject to potential transformation. As I will describe, through tinkering to achieve good eldercare at a distance, kinship and gender are enacted in new ways, too.

Looking at how migrating female nurses participate in enacting care for their parents remotely, I discovered that their parents expect them to call home more often than sons (chapter 4), but also that their other duties have shifted from marrying early to migrating abroad, sending remittances, and visiting their parents regularly. To show how this shift has occurred and what it entails, it is first necessary to describe the position of Syrian Christian women, especially in relation to the conventional ethics of eldercare in Kerala.

DOWRY AND INHERITANCE

Syrian Orthodox Christian women belong to the "dominant minority" of those of upper-caste and now often middle-class background, although they are often still marginalized as women in a patriarchal society (Thomas 2018, 6). Syrian Christians follow patrilineal kinship, including the practice of patrilocality, within the "matrilineal ethos" of Kerala where matriliny was historically present until its official abolishment in the nineteenth century (de Jong 2011). Tracing kinship through female or male line, of course, does not automatically imply that either women or men, respectively, have all power in their hands. As Robin Jeffrey (2004, 648) has noted in her description of matriliny in Kerala, "though the families were based on mother's homes and organized through the female line, the controllers and decision makers were men." Nevertheless, such historical context has empowered Syrian Christian women to challenge patriarchy in some ways. One example is the legislation of equal inheritance for daughters and sons, which Mary Roy achieved almost single-handedly (Philips 2003). Despite this remarkable triumph—or perhaps precisely because she dared to challenge the conventional way of living—she was reviled among some people I met in Kerala. One couple, for example, agreed that she was a "scandalous woman" who got divorced and then demanded inheritance although she had already received her share in the form of dowry.

Although legally prohibited in India since 1961, dowry, or *stridhanam* in Malayalam, is a persistent practice whereby the bride's family transfers property, large sums of money, and other "gifts" such as cars to the groom's family (Das Gupta et al. 2003; Diamond-Smith, Luke, and McGarvey 2008; Philips 2003). In fact, Kerala has seen the sharpest inflation of dowry in the past several decades and has the highest average dowry among all Indian states (Anukriti, Prakash, and Kwon 2021). Based on an analysis of 40,000 marriages in rural India, by 2008 the average net dowry in cash had reached 50,000 Indian rupees (about 700 U.S. dollars) among Christians and Sikhs and INR 30,000 (USD 400) among Hindus. This is

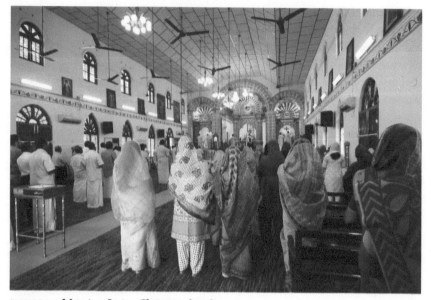

FIGURE 5.1. Mass in a Syrian Christian church.

in addition to about INR 40,000 (about USD 550) worth of other material contributions and the cost of the wedding itself (Anukriti, Prakash, and Kwon 2021).[1] These, at least, are the official figures.

One fine Sunday, I joined a morning mass in a church near Kottayam. I stood at the back of the church on the right side, behind other women of all ages who had raised the upper parts of their colorful saris or shawls over their heads (figure 5.1). The floor was covered in a soft brown carpet with a hypnotic pattern, which gave me a feeling of being swept toward the altar. A red runner rug separated the church space in two parts: women stood to the right of it, and men to the left. Most of the male congregation wore *mundu dhotis*, as the traditional south Indian white cotton cloth with a golden rim is called. Here, under the swishing sound of ceiling fans, I learned that the priest's announcements of weddings after the mass were accompanied by public declarations of the amount of dowry, of which 10 percent would be transferred to the church. A later conversation with a priest revealed that dowry amounts were often much higher than those reported in the press, raising to cash transfers as high as several *lakhs* (1 lakh is INR 100,000 or about USD 14,000) and up to 1 *crore* (100 lakhs, or about USD 140,000).[2]

Related to inheritance, stridhanam can be considered the woman's share of her father's property; it varies according to the economic class of the family, and it may be higher—but is usually lower—than the share that her brothers receive (Visvanathan 1989). The caveat of such succession is that among Syrian Christians stridhanam is transferred to the father of the husband, rather than the woman herself. The wife can therefore only start to enjoy her stridhanam when it is gifted from her father-in-law to her husband in the form of property and house-building materials at the birth of her first child (Visvanathan 1989, 1343). This system of inheritance has been challenged through legislation instituting the right to equal inheritance, yet the impact of this rule on the empowerment of women remains unclear. Despite its revolutionary character, the new succession law is effective only when the male head of the household dies without leaving a will (Chacko 2003). Even when that happens, women still tend to waive inheritance claims on property out of loyalty to their male relatives (Philips 2003).

In discussing the position of women in Kerala, Praveena Kodoth, a professor specializing in gender at the Centre for Development Studies in Thiruvananthapuram, told the *Indian Express* (Varma 2021),

> Dowry is just the symptom of a larger problem and the larger problem is marriage. The problem is that a woman is not seen as having a life if she's not married. In Malayalam, they say, "Ninakku oru jeevitham vende?' (Don't you need a life?). What does that mean? They say phrases like, "Ozhinju poyi, ninnu poyi, irunnu poyi" (goes away, got left behind, got sat behind) if you are not married which means you don't move. They don't say that about men. . . . [3]
>
> Another aspect is that women are not seen as moving to enter the labor market as men are. Even when families think of educating their girls, they think differentially about what they are going to do with this education. Lots of families think if a girl has the kind of job that doesn't threaten the marriage, then that's fine. Like a teacher, nurse, or a nine to five clerical job, that's not bad, but let's say a sales person or someone who has to travel. . . .
>
> A woman's income may be important, but it's always seen as supplementary, like a second income that can be compromised subject to ifs and buts. All of this is part of the problem of dowry. You (women) don't have that earning capacity and need protection. So the girl has to come in with some kind of property.

As Kodoth pointed out, limited possibilities for mobility or choice of profession, depending on family approval and coupled with discriminatory wages, lead to low bargaining power for women within their households. According to a 2017–2018 government report on gender, Kerala has the highest female unemployment rate in India, with 14 percent unemployment among women compared with 3 percent among men. Furthermore, men have higher average salaries than women in almost all employment categories (Babu et al. 2019).

The balance in "bargaining power" (Agarwal 1997), however, has improved to a certain degree in those households in which women engage in international female labor migration. I am not alone in making this argument: Sheba George

(2005), Marie Percot (2012), and Ester Gallo (2006) have made this same point in their work on migrant female nurses in the United States, Ireland, and Italy, respectively. All three scholars described the troubled position of men who join their wives abroad, where they often fail to find employment that comes close to their wives' wages. These "nurse-husbands" (George 2005), a derogatory term indicating their economic dependence on their wives, often assume caring responsibilities for their children and perhaps find work in occasional or part-time low-skilled jobs such as social work and domestic care.

In the U.S. Keralite diaspora, one realm that the nurses' husbands have preserved for themselves is the Syrian Orthodox Church. As George (2005) has described, organizing activities and assuming leadership roles within the church are the men's domain and have become the most important means for men to uphold their social status, personal respect, and patriarchy at large. Further, resistance to women's gains in bargaining power can be observed in the popular discourses describing migrating female laborers. To offer but a couple of examples, the movie *Kadal Kadannu Oru Mathukkutty* (Ranjith 2013) presents female nurses working abroad as bossy and dominating their husbands, and *Life of Josutty* (Joseph 2015) shows migrating nurses as unfaithful and neglectful of their kinship obligations. They are portrayed not only as bad wives but also as bad daughters-in-law and poor congregants.

Money, then, is intricately implicated in enacting Malayali women as subordinated members of society through both the dowry and inheritance systems. Through money flows within those systems, a woman's identity is established and maintained as one that is subject to her relationships with her male kin as husbands, fathers, and brothers. The importance of money in keeping women in their position becomes evident whenever the systems are challenged, as demonstrated by the equal inheritance law and through international labor migration whereby women become the main breadwinners in the household.

Money, then, can also serve to challenge the established patriarchal practices. The women who draw on it to contest the conventional dowry and inheritance systems are often met with resistance. One way in which this plays out is in the field of morality, as women like Mary Roy and migrating nurses become portrayed as "bad." In what follows, however, I show that these nurses and their families have developed a different understanding of international migration, namely as a practice of eldercare. This framing helps them preserve their moral position as good daughters.

In this process of transformation of women's roles and status—indeed, their social identity—through care practices, money is involved in the form of remittances. To understand the significance of this shift, the next section illuminates the established moral conventions of good eldercare in Syrian Christian families as they are tied to the expectations toward women as wives, daughters, and daughters-in-law.

SYRIAN CHRISTIAN ETHICS OF ELDERCARE

As we waited for his students to complete an assignment, I took the opportunity to ask their teacher, Jacob, a Syrian Christian himself, if he thought that the different religions in Kerala influenced people to take care of their parents in different ways. He nodded without giving it a second thought. According to Jacob, there was a certain "fear that is instilled in people by the church." He added that it was the "duty of Christians" to take care of parents; otherwise, their reputation as good Christians would suffer. During mass, priests would preach that people will receive in their own old age the kind of treatment they were giving their parents. Jacob's words reminded me of the memes on eldercare and abandonment that traveled around on social media (chapter 3).

In this context, how do children provide good care for their parents? Like in other patriarchal religious communities across India, filial obligations differ for sons and daughters among Syrian Christians. Sons are expected to provide for their parents financially and through co-residence, but the main filial duty for daughters is to marry and to do so as early as possible (Percot and Rajan 2007). Across the country, in 2015–2016, the average age for women at marriage was 18 years in rural locales and younger than 20 years in urban environments. Women who have higher education, come from wealthier families, and have a Christian religious background marry slightly later, between 21 and 23 years of age (International Institute for Population Sciences 2017).

After marriage, daughters belong to their husband's family and should provide care for their parents-in-law; simultaneously, they are discharged from care obligations toward their own parents. Susan, a middle-aged nurse studying for the International English Language Testing System (IELTS) test after her husband's failed stint in the Gulf, provided a telling example. One Monday afternoon after class, I accompanied her to the public library just around the corner from the English language school. Tall trees on the side of the path protected us from the sun, making for a pleasant stroll. Inside the yellow three-story building, dotted with air conditioning condenser units, Susan returned an English novel and picked out a new one for herself to enjoy, while I browsed through used books whose pages had turned brown with time (figure 5.2).

On our way back toward the main street, we passed a foundation stone marking the spot where later that year, in May 2015, a magnificent sculpture would be unveiled. Akshara Silpam, as the thirty-two-foot (almost ten meters) high sculpture was named, portrays a mother initiating her children into the world of letters. Its main message, the library website notes, is that "a child should learn the alphabet from the Mother, getting the maternal touch and care from its tender age, and that protects it from drifting on to wrong tracks in later life."[4] Coincidentally, this was where Susan told me of the shocking change in her mother's attitude toward her at the time of her marriage.

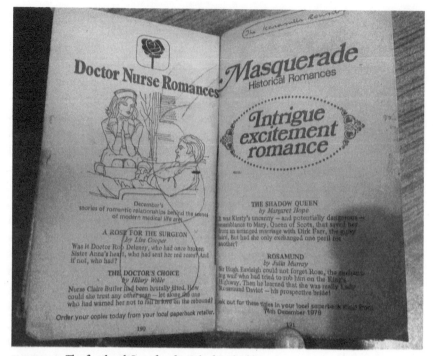

FIGURE 5.2. The first book I randomly picked in the library.

After Susan's wedding, her mother, with whom she had been exceedingly close during childhood, suddenly changed her behavior toward her, saying that Susan was no longer a part of her natal family. More than two decades after the event, Susan's voice and eyes still displayed outright disbelief that her relationship with her own mother changed so dramatically, and almost overnight. Although her mother's attitude was difficult for Susan to accept, it was in accordance with the general expectations of her environment: a daughter's bond with her natal home is severed at marriage, and she becomes a part of her family-in-law, including through caring for her husband's parents (see also Trawick 1990, 163).[5]

The rupture of the parents-daughter bond is linked to the practice of patrilocality; it is generally considered inappropriate for parents to live with their daughters (Bailey, Hallad, and James 2018, 8; Gallo 2005, 230). As life does not neatly follow socially prescribed norms, there are of course exceptions, but they are rare and so only prove the rule. During my fieldwork, I met only one family where a married couple with children lived with the wife's parents, but this arrangement took several years of discussions, and it stirred quite some tension among the family members.

Several years after walk to the library, Vasu, a progressive priest who fervently challenged common gender roles, explained to me through a lengthy exchange of audio messages on WhatsApp that patrilocality and the idea that women should exclusively provide hands-on care only to their parents-in-law was supported by the church:

> Girls are sent to their husband's house at marriage, and then they should take care of their husbands' parents, not their own parents. For example, if a wife asks the priest, "Please pray for my father and mother, they are a bit sick," then the duty of the priest should be to say, "Why don't you stay with your parents for a week?" But he doesn't say that. Instead, he says, "Ok, I will pray for you." That's it! I think the response should be, "Why don't you spend some time with your own parents, taking care of them?" But unfortunately, that is not what I heard from many priests because the family of her parents doesn't belong to their parish! A priest just needs to care for those around him, not the people like a wife's parents who belong to another parish.

According to conventional practices, a wife's visits to her parents should be approved by her husband and parents-in-law. As Susan Visvanathan (1989, 1343) writes of marriage rules among Syrian Christians, "marital discord may result from too frequent return to the natal household, and the bride has to contain her anxieties about her parents ageing and their state of health since these are in a strongly patrilineal society not her concern, but that of her brothers and their wives." In practice, evidently things are not always so clear-cut; some Syrian Christian priests strictly implement traditional gender roles while others, like Vasu, challenge them. Further, as I show later in this chapter, through gaining income women may gain bargaining power to negotiate more frequent visits to their parents.

BEING A GOOD DAUGHTER-IN-LAW

"I took such good care of my mother-in-law," said Hannah, a schoolteacher in her 40s, when I asked her to describe the last time her mother-in-law had been sick. We were sitting in the spacious, tranquil court of the Ayurvedic hospital where I was staying as a guest and she was waiting for her treatment. When her mother-in-law suddenly became ill, Hannah took leave from her work. During that time, she provided hands-on care for her mother-in-law, which was no small task. "How long did it all last?" I asked her. "A month?"

> No, only a week. But that week felt like two, three months to me. So much work, my goodness! Hardly any space to breathe . . . Mommy was hospitalized twice. If she wanted to eat something specific while in the hospital, she would tell me, and I prepared it according to her taste.
> The second time she came back from the hospital she could not move. I realized she was really very sick because she would not eat anything; she just had the

medicine, and she would not even know what medicine she was eating. Then I got really scared because she was panting for breath. So I started giving her food, but she only ate one teaspoon at a time. That is all that she had. People said to give her milk, so I gave her milk, for calcium.

I persevered, and she slowly started gaining her health, and then in about one week she was better. In that way I took real good care. I always changed her clothes, I gave her a sponge bath, I made sure that I put powder on her body, whatever I knew I should be doing, that's what I did. She also told me what to do, so it was easy for me. Otherwise, I would just count the stars because I don't know anything about taking care.

Hannah laughed at her own metaphor.

Yeah, I would really count the stars! If I had to go out somewhere, a maid we hired would be there with my Mommy. See, she was not aware of anything, who was taking care of her, who was by her side. When I gave her food, she stared at me, wondering, "Who is this?" It was very bad because of all the medicines and all the pain. She was unable to sit up. I literally had to take her, lean her on my chest and my shoulder, and I was feeding her.

Then, it was very hot during that time, so she got a skin rash. Even though I took that much care! The skin was peeling off. Oh, my goodness! Seriously, in spite of me taking that much care! And I left it open, not covered in clothes. I put on the fan, and I put ice on the rash, and then I cleaned it properly with powder, and within two days she was fine, and I put her clothes back on. See, I decided I'm not going to make my mother-in-law—or whoever it is—die with all that smell. So now she cannot live without me. People started saying how much I took care of her.

I could see in Hannah's face that she was quite proud of herself. After a brief pause she continued,

When she was in the hospital, Daddy was taking care of her there, and I had to stay at their home because of the dogs. They won't eat food just like that. They're very neat, you must clean the kennel, maybe wash the kennel, then we need to prepare the food then and there and give it to them. They are very choosy. When I had to go home for a week, Daddy took over, and they would not eat. When I returned to their house, the dogs had become so lean! I felt so bad that I did what I did. Then I made chicken soup, I put a little extra rice, I gave it to the dogs, and by the time I returned to my home, Mommy was OK, and the dogs were healthier.

Hannah laughed again.

And then, I cooked food for Daddy. Timely food. And he's very choosy, too. I had to cook maybe three times a day. What else did I do? I had to keep the house clean, so Mommy could be at peace because the house was in good hands. I was running around and cleaning constantly. See, she doesn't like the place untidy. And then the constant visitors, they kept coming, and I had to attend to them as well.

"Why were they coming?" I asked.

To see how she was. It always happens here. There were times when I did not open the door. That would be the time Mommy was sleeping, so I would not want anybody to disturb her. At times Daddy would leave the door open, and people just walked in. Once I heard a whole family there! Some seven or eight people, and I told them to leave; otherwise, she would never get to sleep. Besides, when visitors came, Mommy would start crying, and I didn't like that. So afterwards I did what calmed her down—I prayed with her."

Hannah provided a wonderful example of what care for older people entails, particularly when their health fails. Her narrative shows very clearly what it means to be a good daughter-in-law and what is considered good eldercare: it includes nurturing a wounded, sick physical body by feeding, bathing, changing clothes, attending to rashes, and chasing away visitors so that the body could rest and recover. But it is also much more than that. Practices like praying together to bring peace after emotional distress are just as important (see chapter 6). Further, those around the sick person must be taken care of as well; Hannah's father-in-law had to be fed too, and the visitors served. The food must be prepared according to everyone's taste, whether they are people or pets, and undertaking all of this can be a rather demanding task. Specifically in relation to food, care is in the application of "kitchen ayurveda," the knowledge of how foods can be used for healing purposes, which is generally passed down from the mother-in-law to her daughter-in-law (Visvanathan 1999). In Hannah's story, the kitchen was undoubtedly "a site of care" (Yates-Doerr and Carney 2016).[6]

Furthermore, by tidying the house and making sure her mother-in-law's dogs were clean and healthy, Hannah attended to what her mother-in-law found important. In this way, the mother-in-law did not have to worry about anything and could focus on healing. Hannah did the same on another occasion when her father-in-law was hospitalized. At that time, she got her hands dirty by picking pineapples from the family plantation. Work on the plantation was more suitable for a man, but Hannah's husband refused to do it. Hannah did not enjoy the work and found it difficult to do, but she stood in for her father-in-law because doing what was usually his task was a part of taking care for him. Many of the practices that Hannah described were thus not directly related to health, yet they contributed to it in significant ways (see also chapter 6).

When I asked her about the involvement of her husband in the practical care for his parents, Hannah laughed and said that "he was always busy with his job. And I told him, 'Right, and I'm jobless!'" While her husband used his job as an excuse, Hannah could not refuse to take care of her parents-in-law. Neither, it seemed, would she want that. She confessed that, although caring was often difficult and not particularly enjoyable for her, she was "happy that God gave her the opportunity" to provide care for her parents-in-law. Through caring, Hannah showed her dedication and humility, and it was not for nothing that "people" recognized her efforts. She was praised as a good daughter-in-law publicly, within and beyond her immediate household, and this increased her status in her community and her feelings of confidence and self-esteem.

AUTOMATIC ATTACHMENTS

Whenever I had no other plans while in Kottayam, I visited the English language school and inevitably I would discover something interesting there because the classroom was packed with nurses who wanted to go abroad. The school was also a fun place to be at around lunchtime. I was always able to sit down with the students, who readily shared with me their homemade rice, fried fish, curd and beans, and cabbage curries, neatly packed in tin lunch boxes or wrapped in yesterday's newspapers or in a banana leaf. These were moments of playfulness, jokes were thrown around, and the halls were full of lighthearted din.

One day in February 2015 after such a lunch, I joined a class of seven students, of whom six were female nurses. While the teacher worked individually with the male student, I had the opportunity to talk to the group. All nurses were married, and all but one had previously tried to pass IELTS at least once. I describe the IELTS test and its effects in more detail later in this chapter, but here I want to bring attention to something that made me think about the relationship between daughters and their parents. As I described my research interests to these women, the one who looked the youngest among them suddenly asked, "Is there any discrepancy between girls and boys in caring for their parents?"

Her question surprised me, and I asked her what she thought of this issue. Instead of receiving a reply from her, the women almost sang in unison that there was a difference, no doubt. "Why do you say that?" I wanted to know. "Daughters know better," one of the group said, and then went on:

NURSE: Girls are more attached to their parents, boys go out to play, spend time with their friends, are busy with their work. There are some limitations for girls, like before 6 o'clock they should be at home; otherwise, it is dangerous. For boys it is fine to go out at night, but for girls it is dangerous. The girls absorb more; they try to understand their parents more. They are better in taking care of their social relationships. It will come automatically. You learn from the family.

T. A.: And what happens when women go abroad? Do they take care of their parents financially?

NURSE: When they go abroad, daughters don't necessarily care for their parents financially, although it also happens today in some families. Nowadays women abroad earn a lot, and they can give a certain amount also to their own parents. But after marriage this is not compulsory.

T. A.: So why do it at all, if it is not compulsory?

NURSE: We feel some responsibility towards them.

T. A.: Why did you say the daughters take care emotionally, but not financially then?

NURSE: When we marry, there are some restrictions from the husband and his family regarding where the money goes, and a wife should give her salary to her husband. But there are no restrictions about who to care for emotionally.

T. A.: Do sons also care emotionally?

NURSE: Yes, they do care, but they spend less time with the parents, that is the difference. They are engaged in their own world, they are busy, they live in their own world.

T. A.: And women are not busy?

NURSE: They are, but they find time for the parents; no matter how busy they are, they always find the time.

From my conversations with many other daughters and sons I learned that emotional attachment to parents was not exclusive to women. Many sons, too, expressed great concern for their aging parents and they were actively involved in their transnational care collectives (see chapters 4 and 6). Yet the talk of intense emotional relationship between daughters and their parents, especially mothers, arose time and again in my conversations in the field (see also Rastogi and Wampler 1999). As one female student in our group conversation said, daughters develop deep emotional attachments to their parents "automatically" through spending more time with them.

After marriage, daughters' visits to their natal home may be regulated by their in-laws, but nobody can tell daughters about how to feel about their own parents even after marriage. Women were considered—by themselves and others—more emotional than men, and therefore naturally more inclined to provide care to aging people. As another person told me, "There is a kind of motherly nature in females that makes them do all these things, provide care, a bit more seriously than males." This assumption underlaid the shaping of new filial obligations for daughters in transnational care collectives.

THE FILIAL DUTY TO FLY

Given the complexity of eldercare practices and their dependence on physical proximity, as Hannah's narrative illustrated, what happened with care for aging people in those families where women migrated abroad as nurses? In chapter 3,

I showed that migrating children were often accused of abandoning their parents out of their own individualistic and materialistic ambitions. Here, I argue that this was not exactly the case. Instead, I found that within transnational collectives care was reconfigured, such that new practices replaced those that were not possible anymore because of the geographic distance among family members. Without clear conventions in place, families tinkered with different sociomaterial arrangements to establish how to carry out care at a distance such that it could still be considered good (chapter 4). In this endeavor, migration was reconceptualized from an act of abandonment to a care practice. In this process, digital technologies but also money played an integral role.

To understand how migrating abroad could shape what it means to be a good daughter—or in other words, how gender and kinship became enacted in new ways through a reconfiguration of filial duties within transnational care collectives—it is important to recognize the involvement of parents in the migration process. Among many families I encountered, parents steered their daughters toward nursing from a young age, and this choice of profession was commonly taken with international migration in mind (see also Nair 2012; Nair and Percot 2007; Percot 2016). In one family, the parents encouraged all three daughters to become nurses and migrate. Their efforts were successful: at the time of my fieldwork, the eldest two daughters had settled in the United Kingdom while the youngest one, Mary, was preparing to follow them (see chapter 4). For that, she only needed to pass the IELTS examination, and she was attempting to do so for the third time.

Mary was a young woman in her mid-20s; her dark hair reached to her waist, but she was more outspoken than most other young female nurses I met. When I pointed that out to her, she laughed and said that her mother really wished she was a boy. As she was growing up, her sisters treated her in that way, too. Within days of knowing me, she invited me to visit her home. After traveling by bus on the main road for a while, we took several turns from one narrow unpaved street into another. Once at her home, Mary briefly introduced me to her parents and then showed me around. At the back of the house was a garden where Mary's father grew spinach and other vegetables, and there was a shed where he kept his gardening and repair tools. Next to their property was a plot of land that they had to sell to finance Mary's eldest sister's nursing studies; the area was big enough for the buyers to build a new house on it. Once in the United Kingdom, Mary's sister had been able to finance a renovation of her ancestral home, which now had three bedrooms, a kitchen, and a room that served as a living and dining room.

Mary's mother was especially engaged with her daughters' careers and migration pathways. Soon enough, she was asking me "how was Switzerland?" Instead of providing an answer, I asked her why she wanted to know about that specific country. She answered mockingly, "Because I heard the flowers there were beautiful!" Seeing the puzzled look on my face, she realized that I genuinely had no idea what she was talking about, and she explained, "I heard the wages for nurses were higher there than elsewhere." It became clear that she considered Switzerland a potential destination country for Mary. And so I realized that although young women had their own individual motivations to pursue work abroad, such as gaining professional and personal experience, international migration was not an individual decision but a "family project" (George 2005, 43; Percot 2016). As I discovered through my further fieldwork, how independent nurses were in making decisions about migration was often related to their family's economic background: the lower their class, the greater the family encouragement for at least one of the children to "fly."[7]

Parents were heavily involved financially in the entire project of their daughters becoming successful nurses who could earn well abroad (see also Gallo 2005, 229). This started with financing the daughters' education, first in nursing and then in the English language. The cost of nursing education has risen in recent years, with the average tuition fees reaching INR 70,000 to 100,000 (approximately USD 1,500 to 2,100) per year at the start of my fieldwork (Johnson, Green, and Maben 2014, 12).[8] Families could thoroughly deplete their savings paying high college fees; in these cases, parents took loans from banks, relatives, or acquaintances (Osella and Osella 2008, 156–160; Percot 2016). One family I met borrowed money for this purpose from their wealthier neighbors, and several nurses mentioned that their families had taken out education loans, which came with steep interest rates. Then parents funded the migration process, another costly and lengthy endeavor. To migrate to English-speaking countries, nurses had to pass the IELTS examination. Fees for language classes and the exam represented additional costs. Finally, the expenses of obtaining visas, travel costs, and perhaps engaging a migration agency would add another INR 100,000 to 200,000 (USD 1,400–2,800) to the bill, according to the people I talked to.

For the lower-middle-class families of small-scale farmers, shopkeepers, and clerks, from which the nurses usually originated, the financial burden of supporting their daughters migration was considerable (Johnson, Green, and Maben 2014). The nurses and their parents mentioned borrowing money, working hard to generate savings, engaging nurses' siblings to help financially, and even selling property as acts of great "sacrifice" on the part of parents. The nurses I met regularly reported that their parents "struggled" and "suffered a lot" to support their migration. Such linguistic expressions were related to their religious background, as idioms of suffering and sacrifice are embedded in Syrian Christianity.[9]

In the Eucharist, a central Syrian Christian liturgy, "gift and sacrifice are inextricably interwoven"—the birth of the Christ was a gift, and his moral life was sacrificed through crucifixion (Visvanathan 1999, 173). This resonates with the affective and material exchanges between parents and their migrating daughters. "Suffering" transpired as a way of doing sociality, which "created a strong sense of belonging to specifically those persons who were the greatest source of the suffering [and] gave children a strong sense of responsibility towards their parents"

(Bomhoff 2011, 132). By contributing to parental suffering, money played an essential part in enacting migration as a new filial obligation for daughters. In line with the special attachment that daughters reportedly had with their parents, the idiom of suffering emotionally tied the daughters to parental reciprocity, which also had to be fulfilled in specific ways. In this context, for daughters to be considered good, they had to find employment abroad and send remittances back home.

To fulfill their duty of migrating for work, nurses generally first sought employment in English-speaking countries where salaries are high and where it is possible to obtain permanent residency. From there, they would be able to regularly send remittances to their parents and secure a stable financial future for themselves and their parents. This path, however, was not always easy to follow. Migration depended greatly on the receiving country and its policies toward migrant labor. In English-speaking countries, one of the most important criteria for a working visa was good knowledge of the English language, as reflected in the results of English language tests such as IELTS.[10] For a working visa in countries such as the United Kingdom, United States, Canada, Australia, and New Zealand, the applicants had to pass each of the four modules (listening, reading, speaking, and writing) of IELTS with at least grade 7.0 on a 9.0 grading scale.

By contrast, countries like Oman had much lower requirements regarding language skills. This was obvious from the job advertisements I found in newspapers and online: the ads for the United Kingdom specified the required IELTS score while those for Oman only stated the years of professional experience necessary to apply. Language requirements, however, may change through time: in December 2018, the United Kingdom lowered the required IELTS grade in writing to 6.5, a change specifically addressing international nurses and midwives (Medacs Healthcare 2019).

IELTS is therefore a classification system that is at once material and symbolic (Bowker and Star 2000). According to the grade received in the IELTS test, Malayali nurses were assigned a particular place in the world in a geographical and social sense. If they scored well enough, the door to "heaven"—as one male nurse and IELTS student described English-speaking countries—was open to them. The promise was of higher financial remuneration, with all the implications this had for their social status in terms of class, including better marriage options as their worth on the "marriage market" skyrocketed. The lower the grade, the worse were their options in migration-destination countries: not scoring high enough would only enable nurses to migrate to places such as the Gulf countries, the Maldives, or Guyana where the salaries were relatively low.

A good daughter had to demonstrate her dedication to the family migration plan by attempting to pass the IELTS exam until she succeeded, which among those with whom I spoke included as many as five attempts. This process could lead to considerable mental stress due to the nurses' feelings of guilt, coupled with social pressure, over their inability to fulfill this new filial obligation. After trying to pass the IELTS exam for several years, one nurse anxiously conveyed that her neighbors and relatives were "starting to ask" why she was still living with her parents rather than moving abroad. A nurse in her situation was expected to migrate at least to a Gulf country, where residency depended on employment and nurses earned substantially more than in India. To illustrate the differences in salaries, one senior nurse reported earning EUR 2,800 (USD 3,200) monthly while working in Malta; a junior nurse said that she received INR 80,000 (about USD 1,200) monthly in Saudi Arabia; another nurse received between OMR 900 and 1,200 (about USD 2,300–3,100) in Oman, based on her experience and length of stay there. By contrast, nurses in Kerala earned about INR 10,000 (USD 150) in 2014.

.   The most recent and trustworthy information about the levels of salaries, the costs of migration bureaucracy, the language requirements, and recruitment events traveled swiftly among the students within the English language school by word of mouth. One day, as I sat with a group of students to work on grammar exercises, one of them mentioned that the British National Health Service (NHS) was about to open interviews for nurses; these interviews were regularly organized in cities such as Kottayam, Kochi, and Delhi. There were five levels of the interview, including a written exam and an oral interview. Such recruiting events were free because they were organized with the support of the local government and paid for by NHS.[11] By contrast, applying for a visa through a recruitment agency was costly and had to be paid out of pocket. Such recruitments were commonly advertised in the local newspapers and on billboards, and potential clients were also enlisted in person around locations where IELTS classes and exams took place. When students went for the exam, people hired by migration agencies reportedly waited outside the examination rooms and tried to talk the students into joining their agency to arrange their migration process.

In the English language school former students often paid visits to Jacob's class. The representation of success by these visitors added to the pressure on current students to succeed in the same way. One day, a young nurse named Anju joined us over lunch "for a visit." Anju had passed the IELTS on her first try and was now working to obtain experience in nursing, which was another common requirement for a work visa. When she arrived, Anju first tried to console one of the girls whose marriage arrangement had been "broken" just before the wedding, reportedly because she had not obtained a high enough score on IELTS. Anju had once been in the same position; her marriage arrangement was unexpectedly broken, but now she was engaged again. She had met her groom-to-be at this very school. Anju then wanted to introduce her fiancé, a tall, friendly looking young man, to Jacob. He was also a nurse and was applying to migrate to New Zealand, while Anju was applying to the United Kingdom. I asked her why they chose to apply for two countries so far apart. "Good question," Anju laughed. The response came from her fiancé: "It's a strategy," he said. "We are trying to get the best deal. If the United Kingdom works for her, I will follow her. If it doesn't work for her, we will have more options if I am applying in New Zealand."

Anju had brought a cake for Jacob, but he said that we, the students and I, should have it. Despite his offer, nobody opened the box, so it was just passed around and then ended up sitting sad and lonely in the middle of the table. Meanwhile, it became clear that Anju's visit had another purpose: she had come to ask Jacob for some advice on how to proceed with her application for the United Kingdom. Jacob turned to Anju's fiancé and warned him seriously not to go to New Zealand because "the sun was dangerous there." Then he added that nurses' salaries were apparently not great there. In Jacob's view, once nurses from India were able to work in Europe, they would have no problem migrating farther afield to the United States or Australia, so he encouraged the couple to focus all their efforts on Europe. "The U.S. is a heaven for nurses," Jacob told me, "because they earn the most there." Although the United States was not recruiting a lot at that moment, Jacob thought that "it will open up again in the next three years, so nurses should go to U.K. now so as to be ready to go to U.S. then."

"How do you know all this?" I asked, surprised at his knowledge and the confidence and trust that he clearly had among young nurses. "I know, that's just how it works," he responded. After all, Jacob had been working in this language school for many years, and most of his students were nurses, so he knew the agenda inside and out. From reports that he received from his former students who regularly dropped by for a visit—and from passionately reading *The Economist*—he had become skilled in following migration trends. He genuinely wanted to help anyone who came to him, and that undoubtedly made him one of the most popular teachers in the school and beyond.

For many nurses, passing IELTS with a specific grade was challenging, and entailed significant costs for English language tuition and multiple test takings. IELTS was commonly a source of frustration because of many months of delays in migration, exacerbated by social pressure from extended family and even neighbors. The pressure was also financial, especially when families were under the burden of loans, including for education. Moreover, passing IELTS with grade 7.0 in all modules became a condition—or an offer—cited in marriage proposals. Unmarried men and their parents were increasingly making this request clear in their marriage advertisements, I was told.[12] Most often, however, this prerequisite was concealed and not known to the potential bride and her parents until she received her IELTS results. If the grades were insufficient for her (and by extension to her future groom) to migrate to an English-speaking country, the marriage proposal might suddenly be broken. As several students of English told me, this could occur indirectly by way of the groom's family unexpectedly demanding a higher dowry that was well above the bride's family's ability to pay.

Flexibility in terms of destination country shows how international migration as a filial duty was a "practical accomplishment" (Winance 2007) that was achieved through tinkering with IELTS scores, migration regimes, and marriages. But if nurses failed to migrate abroad for whatever reason, I was told that at least some parents would "stress them" about it, telling them that they were "irresponsible" and "not caring" toward them and their own (future) children. These nurses would seek an alternative solution, which often involved internal migration. Thus, the last and least desirable option would be to find employment in another Indian state, preferably in a city such as Mumbai or Delhi where salaries for nurses were reportedly higher than in Kerala, at around INR 25,000 (USD 370) monthly.

Failure to migrate internationally could result in mental and financial struggles for the whole family and could even have tragic ramifications. A notorious example was Beena Baby, a nurse who committed suicide after her "inhuman treatment" as an employee of a Mumbai hospital (*Hindustan Times* Correspondent Mumbai, 2011). Her fate resonated with nurses across India who received salaries that were too low to repay their educational loans, while their employers prevented them from migrating by withholding their professional certificates (Timmons, Evans, and Nair 2016, 44). Beena Baby's suicide sparked numerous protests, which led nurses to self-organize into what later became the United Nurse Association. In April 2018, after years of protests, the Kerala government raised the minimum monthly wage for nurses to INR 20,000 (about USD 290) with significant backlash from health-care institutions (*Express* News Service 2018; TNM Staff 2018).

Money in the form of investments in nurses' education was thus involved in enacting international migration as a new duty of eldercare. This duty was reinforced through the idiom of suffering, activating affect as a mechanism to create a feeling of obligation from children, especially daughters. International migration as a filial obligation involved some flexibility in terms of destination countries, but only to a certain degree. This limitation was contingent on the amount of money that the family invested into the project of migration: the larger the burden of parental suffering, specifically through assuming debt, the greater the pressure on children to successfully migrate and repay the sacrifice through remittances.

SACRIFICING FOR REMITTANCES

Significantly, for female nurses the filial obligation to migrate became more important than the duty to marry early. Migrant nurses generally did not marry before the age of 25, three years later than the average for Christian women in Kerala and five years later than all Keralite women (Percot and Rajan 2007, 321). This delay created "a window of opportunity," as one nurse told me, laughing. During the years between finishing studies and marrying, daughters could earn a salary to "repay the suffering" of their parents via remittances, as several explained, without potential restrictions imposed by in-laws. In this way, another new filial obligation came to enact good daughters within transnational care collectives: sending remittances to their parents.

By fulfilling this obligation, daughters helped their natal families considerably. For example, as an unmarried nurse in her mid-20s who had been working in the Gulf for a year, Nisha regularly sent almost all her monthly salary to her parents. Her financial contribution to the household sufficed to cover her parents' and younger brother's living expenses because none of them worked; to repay her educational loan; to pay her brother's university fees; and to renovate the family's house. Although Nisha was barely on speaking terms with her father, her remittances paid for his health expenses after his stroke. Besides all this, Nisha was also saving money for her own dowry as was common for migrating nurses.

I visited Nisha's family at their home, in a rural setting outside of Kottayam, with Elia, a young professional who worked in a bank, as my interpreter. Nisha's single-story house, surrounded with a garden and tall rubber trees, was freshly repainted. On the outside it was bright pink, and on the inside the light blue shade of the walls matched well with the wooden flooring. There were still painting buckets in the corner of one room. Nisha's mother, a small woman with a wrinkled face, wearing a black and white nighty, explained that they wanted to renovate the house further, enlarge it even, but they would do it later.

Nisha's father, wearing a white shirt and a red and blue checkered lungi, sat on a plastic chair in the corner of the sitting room while Nisha sat on a cushioned bench across from me. The main door made a kind of a fence between the two of them. Without saying a word, he brought an extra fan in the room and pointed it at Elia and me. Later, Elia and I discussed how fathers would commonly quietly disappear from the house whenever I visited, and Elia said that such behavior was quite typical. Fathers were "the head of the family," and they probably did not want to show their ignorance—they could not speak English well, so they preferred to leave. Nisha's father had remained in the room, but during the conversation that followed, Nisha's mother had the most to say.

As soon as we sat in the car again, pulling off the driveway, Elia mumbled in a low voice, "Typical family." "What do you mean?" I asked, astonished.

Remember when you asked the mother why it was so important for her to know that Nisha was doing well abroad? She replied that she was concerned about her daughter, yes, but her initial response was actually that the daughter needed to be healthy to keep working! Then, when asking about what the mother wished for her daughter, she said, "To find a good husband who would allow her to keep supporting us."

The girl gets 80,000 rupees [around USD 1,000] a month in the Gulf, of which she sends 70,000 rupees [over USD 900] home. That's an enormous amount! And where does that money go? Nisha's own education loan needs to be paid off, the interests are high on it, and as she couldn't repay it while studying, so that is about 4 to 5 lahk [US$5,300–6,600]. Then she is paying for her brother's education for which they are not taking a loan. She is paying for all the expenses in the house as neither her mother or father have any work, she's paying for health expenses, as her father had a stroke. Then think of the house renovation, the computer, and now they're starting to plan her wedding. Nisha has started buying gold, and for that she asked permission from her mother!

She's paying for her brother's study fees, too. But once he grows up, he will most likely forget all about his sister's help. He will be the treasure of the family, and she will be treated as if she has never even been there. So she might end up hurt and disappointed. I just hope the girl will not get cheated.

Elia's assumptions were not completely ungrounded. I came across multiple examples of families in which women worked hard, only to pay for their sisters' dowries and their brothers' education. But at the end of the day, when their inheritance was to be divided, the sons typically acquired all the property while the daughters were left with peanuts.

"These daughters, they are nothing but milking cows," Elia firmly concluded. I was struck by this image, and it continued to haunt me. In patrilineal Indian families, daughters have long represented an economic burden to their parents due to the practice of dowry, and many considered spending money on their daughters, for example, by paying for their education, as "investing in another family's daughter-in-law" (Das Gupta et al. 2003, 17). However, in transnational nurse families, this had changed: "the 'burden of having a daughter' . . . turns out much lighter if she is able to get a nursing diploma" (Percot 2016, 256). Even more, due to their ability to send home remittances from abroad, daughters with nursing degrees became an "asset" (George 2005, 42).

Throughout my fieldwork, I never came across any nurse that would complain about migrating, and I did not hear anyone use the expression about milking cows again. Quite on the contrary, most nurses were satisfied of their decision to migrate; they were happy and proud to be able to help their families in Kerala (see chapter 6). Additionally, they emphasized the benefits of migration for them and their own children. As I describe later in this chapter, many made it clear that they were abroad not only for their parents, but also to ensure their own pensions and support the education of their children, so they were investing in their future, too. In contrast to Nisha who was still young and unmarried, the nurses I met in Oman, who were married and in their 50s, assumed more control over their money and how they spent and distributed it. Despite not enjoying the same privileges as the local population, they found ways to enjoy themselves. Even among those who did not have their family nearby, many appreciated their relative freedom from some obligations, such as attending countless social events, that come with being embedded in the thick social network in Kerala.

It is impossible to establish the degree to which any nurse may have been pressured into migration and into sending remittances. One thing is evident, however: the decision to migrate was generally not entirely their own because this process required a great deal of investment in terms of time, finances, and emotions from the whole family. The idioms of parental sacrifice and suffering commonly played a role in emotionally tying children, particularly daughters, to their new filial obligations of migrating abroad and sending home remittances. When complying, such children were also referred to as good children by their parents, those around them, and even themselves. "Yes, I am buying all the phones and everything for my parents," one male nurse told me with a sense of pride in his voice. "See, I'm a good son!" he added and laughed.

The stories of nurses from Kerala and their families indicate that good care is a matter of making certain decisions, with contingent sacrifices. They also shed light on broader questions of care: could some practices still be considered as enacting care if they were undertaken out of compulsion rather than genuine concern? To what extent does one sacrifice oneself to provide good care for others, in this case one's parents? Some insight on this comes from Vasu, a priest I interviewed about what it meant to be a good son or daughter within the Syrian Christian ethics:

You might have heard about this Biblical statement, "Love your neighbor as you love yourself." It's the most misunderstood statement, I think. Everyone is talking about loving your neighbor. But that sentence is meaningful only with the other part—as you love yourself. That means, first you need to love yourself. First you need to know yourself. Respect and accept who you are and what you are. Only then you can love your neighbor.

You need to be healthy yourself, only then you can care for others. But unfortunately, in many cases that doesn't happen. Children often love their parents blindly. But when you love your parents, first you need to be healthy to support them, physically, mentally, and emotionally. If you are emotionally unwell, how can you emotionally support your mother or father? If you are physically not healthy, how can you physically lift your mother when she needs it?

I know a nurse from Kerala who lives in Europe. She is blindly supporting her family financially, emotionally, in every way. But she is not physically fit. She is having serious health issues. She shouldn't work every day, her work schedules should be shorter, with less hours. She has told me all about it. Yet she doesn't care about that, and she's doing extra work, overtime, to send that extra money to her family in Kerala, to her parents and parents-in-law. She is trying to be a good daughter, but she is sacrificing her own health for this. Meanwhile, I visit her family often because I sometimes buy things for them on her behalf. They know she is sick, but they say, "Oh, she is young, it's OK." She is now in her late 40s, so ignoring health issues at this age could mean serious consequences for her.

And this is not the only case; you could find many similar examples. It is important to help your family, yes, but first you need to make sure you yourself are well, in every aspect.

Despite remittances being such a significant element of transnational care collectives, receiving money from daughters was a sensitive topic to discuss with parents. Generally speaking, in patrilineal Indian families, parents tend to "incur a considerable loss of respect" if they are cared for, financially or otherwise, by their own daughters (Lamb 2000, 84). In line with that, the parents of female nurses often found it difficult to acknowledge publicly that they were being supported by their daughters. Those who did talk about accepting their daughters' financial contributions justified their actions through idioms of suffering and sacrifice.

For instance, one father firmly declared that he did not want to depend financially on his daughters, so he continued to work himself. His wife, however, emphasized that she and her husband "suffered a lot" for their daughters. She added that while they could "not demand" anything from them, it was perfectly fine to "accept whatever [their] daughters were willing to give."

The practice of daughters sending remittances was thus fraught with "intergenerational ambivalence" (Gallo 2018). Parents could not make open demands on their daughters for remittances or complain if they did not receive any or enough, yet they also depended on their daughters' financial support. Despite the efforts of the Indian government to increase health insurance and pension coverage beyond specific target groups, more than 70 percent of older adults in Kerala depend on their children or other relatives for living and health expenses (van Dullemen and de Bruijn 2015; Zachariah, Mathew, and Rajan 2003, 402). To mitigate the contradiction between their financial needs and the patriarchal stipulations of financial independence from daughters, parents tended to appeal to their daughters' emotions via activating the idioms of "suffering" and "sacrifice" and by "accepting" rather than "expecting" financial support from them. Thus, as sending remittances to their own parents became a new duty for good daughters, the way in which this norm was enacted did not directly confront the patrilineal system.

By migrating abroad, the nurses were not only repaying the sacrifice to their parents, but were also making sacrifices themselves, such as being separated from their spouses and children for various periods of time. Such sacrifice was less heavy if they managed to migrate to a country where they also saw benefits for themselves. When they succeeded in finding employment in a European country or in the United States, United Kingdom, Canada, or Australia, they mentioned a number of reasons for migration other than financial care for their family. Nurses commonly told me that the "standard of living" was better in those countries and so were work conditions. Their friends who were already in one of those countries had reported that they were better respected at work, they had greater opportunities for learning and promotion, and the general facilities—from shopping to public infrastructure and education—were seen to be superior to those found in Kerala. Besides, those countries offered generous pensions to which they were entitled upon retiring.

Despite all this, migration could be emotionally challenging even for young nurses in Europe. Pia, for example, migrated to Germany during the COVID-19 pandemic when the need for nurses increased there; however, because the migration procedure was demanding, she had to leave her young daughter in the care of her parents. "It was really very hard for me to cope without my family, but I sacrificed for a bright future, and I hope that I can bring my family to Germany soon," she wrote in a WhatsApp message.

REDISTRIBUTING CARE WORKLOAD

Besides the immediate impact of improving the family's financial situation, the money that nurses earn abroad can help them to marry into a "good family." This indicates a family that is well positioned in terms of class and caste as well as an advance over the social status of their natal family. With a female nurse's marriage, the "window of opportunity" for her parents to receive remittances could close because afterward she should start contributing financially to her in-laws (see also Gallo 2005).

Some parents hoped to reduce this risk through their choice of the groom. Nisha's mother, for example, wanted to find "a good husband" for her daughter, meaning "one that would allow Nisha to keep supporting us after marriage." A "good husband," then, would accept that his wife financially supports her parents. This sort of tolerance was not conventional, but it became a sought-after quality in marriage negotiations. The nurses' in-laws expected their migrating daughters-in-law to share their income with their husbands, call their parents-in-law regularly, and stay with them when visiting Kerala. These practices were in line with the prescribed role of daughters-in-law within the patrilineal system. But the money that the nurses earned increased their bargaining power with their in-laws such that they could negotiate about caring for their own parents as well as meeting their care responsibilities to their new husband's family.

Sara, for example, whose story served as an opening to this book (see chapter 1), had been working and living by herself in Oman for over a decade with the main goal to provide financial support for her husband, children, mother-in-law, and parents in Kerala. This is how she described her obligation to reciprocate her parents' investment in her, rather than focusing exclusively on her in-laws:

> I am giving preference to my parents rather than my in-laws. I am always telling that to my husband, then he tells me, "But your home is here," in his parents' house. Then I say, "No, don't think like that, because if my parents didn't educate me, I would be nothing, I would not get any money ... Because of my parents I got this job. If they didn't educate me, I would not get the chance to migrate. Nothing from your side, no? All support came from my parents. Because of them I got this job. So I have to see them first."

Despite her husband's initial protests, Sara felt deeply obliged to reciprocate to her parents through remittances and also by visiting them when on leave in Kerala. She used the bargaining power she had gained by becoming the family breadwinner to convince her husband, Alvin, that it was the right thing to do. Sara referred to her parents' "struggling" to justify that "all parents, mine and my husband's, are the same" in deserving support from their children. In this way, money helped to establish new norms of intergenerational reciprocity, whereby daughters played a key role in the economic and affective care for their parents as well as parents-in-law.

This was significantly different from the discourse on eldercare that discouraged daughters from financially supporting their parents and from living with them (Bomhoff 2011, 205). Further, this mentality was transferred to the next generation: "Just as my parents sacrificed for me, that's how I am now sacrificing for my children," Sara stated firmly. "Now I am here, I am struggling for them. They must understand that. My husband and I need to forget about our wife–husband relation, for them! So, when they marry, they must also think, 'See, my parents struggled for me, so I cannot forget that.'"

As daughters successfully advocated for sharing remittances and staying with their parents while on leave, these practices also influenced their care workload. Sara described her physical exhaustion from paying attention to her parents as well as her mother-in-law during her yearly visits to Kerala. "When I'm in Kerala, I am mentally ok, but physically I'm not well," Sara told me and smiled. "If I stay at my parent's house one night, I have to stay at my husband's house with him and my mother-in-law the next. So, I alternate like this, traveling every day. Then I tell my husband, 'Oh my god, I want to sleep like in Oman!'" She laughed.

Nevertheless, it would be difficult to claim that for married nurses working abroad the eldercare workload simply doubled. Rather, husbands became active members of their transnational care collectives, too. Within these collectives the care workload became distributed differently in the context of the changing constructions of masculinity, which also increasingly came to include men as child-carers (see also Gallo

2006; Gallo and Scrinzi 2016; Osella and Osella 2006) and, as I show, elder-carers. This shift occurred in tandem with new ways of enacting the norms for good daughters.

Alvin, Sara's husband, was a case in point. Alvin was a lean, humble, and polite man, and when I briefly met him in Kerala, he smiled a lot and spoke softly. He also seemed a bit nervous, perhaps because he was in a hurry to pick up their children from school. He had just enough time to explain that he had joined his wife in Oman for a few years but then returned to Kerala because his mother was alone and not very healthy—she "struggled with breathlessness." So Sara "sent him" to stay with his mother. In this way, Alvin could also take care of their children and Sara's parents. Sara suggested this arrangement to Alvin because she could "make as much money in one month as he would have made in three to four months."

Once in Kerala, Alvin worked on renovating his ancestral home, which he would eventually inherit. He regularly traveled by car between his mother's and his in-laws' houses, which were about two hours apart, taking care of food supplies, house maintenance, and visits to the doctor when needed. Because Alvin had no income of his own, he was unable to take care of his mother financially as a good son would do. Instead, he stood in for Sara by providing practical care to his mother and to his parents-in-law. He said, "I take care of the three of them, because one day we, too, are going to be old" (see chapter 3).

The changes in Sara's and Alvin's eldercare practices reflected their different levels of bargaining power, which were directly linked to their earning (in)abilities shaped by international migration. Alvin's example shows how international migration "opens up new space representing newly emergent assemblages of gender, power, economics and cultural ideals that may put pressure on men to perform their masculinities differently, or at least more flexibly" (Yeoh and Ramdas 2014, 1203). In transnational care collectives with female nurses abroad, men's duties shifted to support eldercare while their role as financial providers decreased. As eldercare practices became reconfigured for daughters and their husbands, the care workload became redistributed in new ways. This enabled family members to continue practicing care, rather than outsourcing it to non-kin from poorer parts of India or the world, as the literature on global care chains describes (Yeates 2012; see chapter 2).

Exploring changes in gender roles in relation to childcare among Sri Lankan transnational families, Michele Gamburd (2008, 23) found that new expectations for migrating mothers and left-behind fathers "reflect the influence of global economy on local social structures." Investigating eldercare practices in transnational care collectives reveals new layers of complexity about gender and kinship. The transformations of the daughter–parent relationship, whereby daughters became primary carers for their own parents through financial, practical, and emotional care, are significant for patriarchal Syrian Christian families in which, just a generation ago, married women had to leave their natal families and focus on their ties with and responsibilities for in-laws (Gallo 2005). The new duties of good daughters conflicted with the Syrian Christian patriarchal practices and beliefs, and so the new care practices I described here were also replete with ambivalence. But rather than openly contesting the conventional way of life, transnational families employed the idioms of parental suffering and sacrifice and talked of accepting rather than expecting financial support from daughters. Moreover, the changes in bargaining power of married daughters remained limited as daughters continued practicing care also for their parents-in-laws, albeit in a different form than in conventional families.

Transnational care collectives were thus established in the context of a complex "geohistory" (Raghuram 2016) of Kerala, influenced by Syrian Christian ethics of eldercare and by patriarchal practices that are common across India, such as the arranged marriage, dowry, patrilineal inheritance system, and patrilocality. Broadening the scope of material semiotics beyond digital technologies showed that within this particular geohistory another nonhuman actor participated in enacting eldercare at a distance: money. For migrating nurses' parents, money in the form of education fees and loans represented an investment, not only to improve the lives of their children and (future) grandchildren but also to support their own eldercare. Their return on investment would materialize through remittances, which were significant against the background of limited social benefits for older adults in India.

Within eldercare practices, an empirical ethics analysis showed, money profoundly influenced the identity of female nurses as good daughters. Through mobilizing affect via idioms of suffering and repaying the sacrifice, money contributed to shifting their filial duties from marrying early to migrating abroad, sending remittances, visiting, and—as I elaborated on in chapter 4—calling home regularly and often more frequently than sons. In the final chapter of this book, I focus again on digital technologies to explore how caring for health and well-being, in particular, is attended to within transnational care collectives.

6 · DOING HEALTH

Care for older adults becomes increasingly complex with time, as the body concedes to the needs and demands of advanced years. Within transnational care collectives of the families I encountered, taking care of health and attending to illness were daily concerns. The parents who were in their 50s and 60s were mostly physically and mentally fit, socially active, including joining religious events, and many engaged in some sort of work, either as shopkeepers, small-scale farmers, or professionals. Many of them, however, had chronic health problems such as diabetes and high blood pressure, and some experienced acute states like food poisoning or fractured bones. Still, they generally were able to manage the practicalities themselves or with the help of neighbors and relatives living nearby.

In this chapter, I explore how health-related situations were attended to within transnational care collectives: what kind of health care was enacted at a distance and through which specific practices? How did digital technologies—and also money—participate in them? What new technologies became included? Who beyond the parents in Kerala and the migrating children became included? And finally, what ambivalences, tensions, and creative solutions arose? I show how phones, photographs, and webcams on smartphones were involved in care practices such as managing chronic illness, responding to health emergencies, and reorienting attention to those who were perceived the most vulnerable during the COVID-19 pandemic.

With age, things tend to change in terms of bodies and minds but also attitudes. If at one point in the family history good eldercare could be reasonably well enacted through the practices of migrating abroad, sending remittances, visiting, and calling frequently (see chapters 4 and 5), an older parent's failing body and mind might put these practices into question as the best care or the kind of good care and caring relationships that the families would wish for. In chapter 5, I wrote about the sacrifices that the parents endure to enable their children to migrate internationally, and the sacrifices that some adult children, especially women who live abroad alone, make through migration. At the end of this chapter, I look at how the families deal with the approaching end of life and yet another kind of sacrifice, which is involved in making decisions about returning to Kerala, either temporarily or permanently, to attend to their parents' ill health. Would the children, by then themselves often entering the second half of their lives, sacrifice work opportunities to be physically near their parents? Or would they sacrifice their career and financial flows and return to Kerala, not only for their relationship with their parents but also in support of the relationships between their own children and their grandparents? What are the ethics of such decisions when they eventually must be made?

Each of the available options, of course, comes with its own consequences that have to be taken into account and be accounted for. As my fieldwork shows, the decisions people make in relation to their migration pathways, departures, and returns reflect and shape who they are as good daughters and sons—hence, these decisions are also an issue of ethics and affect.

TELEMONITORING CHRONIC ILLNESS

Toward the end of February 2014, I climbed into a small van that belonged to an Ayurvedic clinic based south of Kottayam, where I was staying for a few weeks. Madesh, who climbed into the driver's seat, was taking me to visit two of his patients, Achamma and Pathrose, an older couple who had four daughters. One daughter, Teresa, was a nurse living in the United States, another was a nurse working in Kuwait, the third was a teacher in a city about three hours' drive away, and the fourth daughter was married and lived around the corner from her parents' home.

Achamma and Pathrose lived alone in a house with a garden, bordering on railway tracks. In contrast to the villas financed with "nurse money" that I had seen elsewhere, theirs was a modest single-story house with a veranda protected with a *poomukham*, the traditional teak railing. This was where we found Pathrose, sitting comfortably in his reclining chair, also made of teak wood. We could hear Achamma busy in the kitchen, the tin plates and pots clinking against each other. I noticed right away that it was difficult for Pathrose to move because he did not stand up to meet us. But then Achamma, a strong and spirited woman, emerged from the house gloriously, pushing away the door curtain with a wide smile across her face. In a matter of moments, the round rattan table in front of us was covered with plates of fresh, sweet jackfruit, guava, and coffee. Cheerfully chatting away, she noted that her husband was "the quiet one" of the couple. "That's how God makes things—puts one such one such together so they can get along!" she laughed.

Of the four daughters, Teresa lived the farthest away from them in terms of geographic distance, yet Achamma talked mostly about her. She told us that Teresa called them on the phone every day, but they only heard from their daughter in Kuwait once a week. When Achamma suggested renovating their house, Teresa, in contrast to her siblings, readily accepted that they did not want to sell it; instead, she supported her parents' wishes and invested in the renovations. That was why she would inherit the house, Achamma and Pathrose had decided. Despite their having so much affection for Teresa, I was surprised to hear Achamma resolutely say that she would never move with her to the United States. "Look at all the fruits that grow in our garden—jackfruit, mango, coconut! Can you get that in the U.S.? No!"[1]

Achamma gave me Teresa's phone number, and about two weeks later I managed to reach her on the phone. For me, sitting in my tiny rented room in Kerala, it was late in the evening, but for Teresa it was early morning in California. She had arrived home after her night shift when she called me.

"I have just saved a person who had a heart attack," she said, and in her voice I could hear genuine happiness and relief, without pride. Despite having had a hard night, she did not want to schedule a meeting for a future time—she preferred to talk to me immediately. And so we talked for an hour and a half, interrupted only briefly as my landlady rang my doorbell to bring me plate that was generously laden with rice, lentils, cabbage curry, and fried fish for dinner.

Teresa had lived with her own family in the United States for the past eight years, and not a day went by without her calling her parents. She actually called twice a day—before and after her night shift. Through a subscription to Vonage, Teresa could call inexpensively through the internet on their landline phone.[2] The twelve-hour time difference worked perfectly for their transnational care collective because their calls always took place at the same interval, at dusk and dawn. Through our discussion it became clear that Teresa was particularly attuned to her parents' health; her father had Parkinson's disease as well as a chronic skin rash:

> I ask my mother, "Morning, how is dad, where is he sitting?" So I know if he is sitting, where he is sitting, and what he is saying; I know his mood. I ask my mom, "Is there any sign of skin infection on his leg? Is he fine moving the lower leg? How is the temperature? What is the color of the skin?" I always ask my mom all these questions. Then I ask her about the site of the wound. How often is it getting worse? Then I have a picture, oh, that is that. OK. It's that same chronic condition.
>
> Today also my mom was saying my dad has some skin problem on his lower legs, and I told her, "Give him some massage so he will have more circulation to that part. That's all, don't take him to any hospital, they will put him there, and he will get lots of antibiotics, and I don't want him to go for that." I always tell them what to do, which kind of blood test they should do. Then I ask about the report, and I give them directions on how to proceed. I don't want them to go for aggressive medical management; they are in their 80s or 70s, that doesn't make any sense to me. I just want them to be comfortable.

Achamma took care of Pathrose practically, by taking him for laboratory tests, for example, but Teresa was deeply involved in doing health care for both her parents. Her support through the phone was neither exclusively emotional nor was it only a form of communication, but it was very pragmatic, too. By making health care at a distance possible, the phone shaped this transnational care collective in several ways. Through daily updates about the smallest details concerning her father's state, gained explicitly through her mother's descriptions or implicitly through nuances of her father's voice and words, Teresa continuously monitored his chronic illnesses, from his skin problem to his Parkinson's disease. The phone, which affords only the transmission of sound, required that Teresa sharpen her listening skills to be able to read her father's voice. Attentive listening was necessary on the phone to discern nuances in the voice and to interpret the meanings of silence (Baldassar 2008; Genovese 2004). And, although the phone did not afford the transmission of visual images, it allowed for visualization; Teresa was using her mother's eyes to form a mental image of the body she was examining at a distance. In doing so, she built on her professional knowledge as well as the intimate familiarity she had with her parents. Teresa thus used her multilayered knowledge of her parents' situation, including about their health histories, personalities, and the relation between them, to set a diagnosis and "direct" them in treatment at a distance.

But why was it important for Teresa to call home as frequently as twice a day? "In this way, I am always there for them; it makes it possible for me to find out if they have any problems and then to call others around them in case they need any help," Teresa explained. Through frequent calls, she signaled to her parents that her caring "attitude" continued despite geographic distance (see chapter 4). More than that, this allowed her to maintain her parents' trust, which she deemed highly important to ensure that they follow the health-related advice which she provided on the phone.

"Trust is the main thing, they must trust you to do what you are telling them to do," Teresa explained. She contrasted her situation with that of her younger sister, who was a nurse working in Kuwait. Teresa had an impression their parents did not take her sister's health advice as seriously as they took hers. After a moment of consideration, she added, "I know my father very well. I know each word that is going to come out of his mouth, when it means something. And I know what is going on between my parents. That's the way this is working out here, otherwise it would not." To carry out telemonitoring successfully, then, frequent calling was key to maintain the trust and the intimate knowledge of Pathrose's illness and of the relationship between him and Achamma, who was the primary hands-on caregiver within this collective.

Digital technologies were clearly significant to telemonitor chronic conditions across distance. Additionally, monitoring was accompanied by other care practices, such as mobilizing people—kin or non-kin—in Teresa's parents' vicinity to provide practical assistance with health-care technologies. Through a video call via WhatsApp, Aaron, an unmarried nurse working in the United Kingdom and the only son to his parents living in Kerala, shared with me how he was arranging care for his father, who had chronic obstructive pulmonary disease (COPD), through his smartphone:

> My father has a problem with breathing; he is on oxygen support. And my mom is diabetic, type 2, but she's doing well at the moment. I talk to her every day, but with my father it's more difficult. We often have different views on things, so it's hard for me to control him in any way. I told him that they should come here and live with me, that would make everything easier for us, as I'm an only son and there's nobody I can ask for help in Kerala, no brothers. But he firmly said, "No, I'm not coming!"— and that's it. So I manage everything from the U.K.
>
> Fortunately, I have a good job, far better than being a nurse in India, and I'm getting a fairly good salary. This allows me to buy all the equipment needed to support a person with COPD in the U.K., and I send it over to my parents via DHL.[3] Oxygen concentrator, pulse oximetry, all sort of things. Now my house in Kerala is like a small hospital. There are three oxygen concentrators, two DPIs [dry powder inhalers], everything is there.
>
> I'm managing things like that over the phone. I talk and talk and talk to people. I have a few friends back home, and I ask them to help my parents when needed, like with setting up the equipment. I pay them some money for that, maybe 20 to 30 pounds (25–40 U.S. dollars) once in a while, so they are happy. They are not nurses, but they know how to connect the oxygen and so on. It's really not that complicated.

Aaron's struggle with taking care of his father was partially linked to his father's character. In contrast with Teresa's parents, Aaron's father was difficult to convince into following any advice, including the idea to relocate abroad (but see Lamb 2009). Moreover, Aaron was an only child, so he had to be creative with organizing hands-on support for his parents. To attend to Aaron's father's serious chronic condition, the transnational care collective was extended to include new people and even new technologies. Multiple health-care devices had to be bought, shipped, installed, and maintained, and a smartphone allowed Aaron to activate and organize several of his friends around this activity.

Money, again, played a part in the form of small payments because this was the most feasible way for Aaron to reciprocate with his friends at a distance (see chapter 4). But his friends were also made a part of the collective through in-person socializing: "When I'm in Kerala, I just invite them for a drink, we have a kind of a party." Without brothers, Aaron invested time and money into maintaining such non-kin relationships so that he could rely on these friendships for the purpose of enacting health care for his parents when needed. This kind of work is rarely seen as a care practice or as health care, yet it was of critical, probably life-saving importance to Aaron's father, as I describe in the next section of this chapter.

More commonly, to support parents' health care, transnational care collectives included nurses' younger siblings who stayed near or with their parents at least until they had finished their studies. Nurse Meena, whom I met in her apartment on the seventh floor of a magnificent block of flats in Muscat, Oman, told me that this was the case in her family. Meena's parents were still relatively young; her mother Sandra was in her 50s, and her father James in his 60s. But James was not in the best of health—he had "sugar," a term that people commonly used to refer to diabetes. His long-term use of diabetes medicines had triggered other health issues, too. As the only health-care professional in her natal and in-law families, Meena was the first point of contact when health-care related advice was needed: "When having any questions about health, I am the first person my mother would call, because I am the only one in the medical field in my family," Meena told me proudly. "Both from my family and from my husband's family, whatever health problem they are facing, they would call me. They cannot go to the doctor for every small issue, of course, because they live a bit out from any major town."

Meena's experience, I found, was in stark contrast with that of male nurses abroad. Anthony, for example, told me that none of his family members, near or far, would ever consult him on any health issue. When I asked him why he thought that was, he replied, "Because nurses are not doctors. They think we don't know anything, we are far below in the hierarchy." Although I heard such reasoning from some other nurses, too, I suspect that the practice of relatives asking nurses for health advice also depended on gender—my fieldwork showed that female nurses are more easily asked for help than male nurses. In chapter 5, I write about how care is often associated with women as a trait that comes to them almost naturally, and it might be that this outlook influences seeking health advice among family members.

Still, even for Meena there were instances in which her advice through the phone did not suffice. Most disturbingly, James occasionally experienced hypoglycemia—a sudden, dangerously low insulin level in his blood—and Sandra could not manage that alone. He might be sweating a lot, or might feel very weak or be shivering; he could identify the hypoglycemia himself according to such symptoms. But it was difficult to know when exactly this would happen, either during the day or at night. Once, Sandra was unsure whether James was sleeping or had fallen unconscious due to hypoglycemia, so she panicked and woke him up from sleep. Events like this were difficult for Sandra, and she often struggled to sleep out of worry for her husband. "He sleeps at night, I sleep by day," she told Meena once.

Because of James's poor health, Meena's younger brother Aju enrolled at a university nearby although he would have preferred to study in another Indian state. Meena's father had to undergo regular monthly checkups at the local hospital. Meena's parents had a car—yet another nonhuman actor shaping health care for James—but they did not drive. So the person who would usually drive them was Aju or, in case he was not available, his cousin who also lived nearby. "We don't have drivers, we have to drive ourselves," Meena added, implicitly noting her family's class because only wealthier people would be able to hire personal drivers in Kerala.

In enacting health care for parents with chronic illnesses, various new human and nonhuman participants joined the transnational care collective, shaping its dynamic in different ways. Which people, from siblings to friends and drivers, and which material objects, from smartphones to specialized health-care devices and cars, became included (or not) often depended on one of the key actors: money. At the same time, affect was an important underlying "glue" (cf. Vertovec 2004) for the collective. This is illustrated through Teresa's daily calls to her parents and her respecting their wish to keep their ancestral home, which fostered trust in their collective. Affect was mobilized through Aaron's regular partying with friends to uphold a sense of a friendship grounded in mutual respect and reciprocity, with the aim of securing care for his parents in times of need.

Affective ties both stimulate and are strengthened through practices such as daily calling, giving advice over the phone, negotiating co-residence with siblings, and partying with friends. These practices all demand time and energy, yet some of them can be more easily recognized as (health)care practices than others. However, over time these seemingly unrelated things that migrating nurses do, both at a distance and when visiting Kerala, are crucial to enacting health care through transnational care collectives.

ACTION IN EMERGENCY

One day, a couple of years before I met their family, Teresa picked up her phone in California only to learn that her mother had suffered a stroke. Teresa did not think twice about it: she immediately bought a plane ticket to return to Kerala as soon as possible. She arrived four days after the event, and her sister came from Kuwait three days after her. Achamma was lucky because her son-in-law who lived nearby had answered her call for help. He transported Achamma to a hospital in a major city, a road trip that took them almost five hours. They decided to drive so far because the local doctor would only attend to her the next morning, so the family chose to make arrangements for clinical care in Kerala's capital and were on their way immediately.

"When my mother had a stroke," Teresa told me on the phone, "I came and stayed with her for five weeks. A physiotherapist came for a home visit and went through the whole exercise program with me so I could learn how to do it. I helped my mother with that program three, four times a day. By the time I returned to the

United States, she started walking again. I am always there whenever they need me because we can have family leave from work when our parents are in trouble. I always take that if I need to. I was traveling back and forth for around eight or ten times in the past eight years since I've lived in the U.S. I'm only not planning to come this year. Well, if they need, I'll go, but for the moment, it sounds like they are fine."

Whether nurses could return to Kerala to visit their ill parents depended on the circumstances, most importantly in terms of their country of residence. This determined their work conditions, including family leave, but also the costs of the trip and the time it would take to reach Kerala. In the language school I met Ela, a middle-aged nurse who had lived in the United Arab Emirates (UAE) for several years; at the time of our encounter, she was preparing to take the IELTS test to move to an English-speaking country next. During her stay in UAE, Ela's mother was diagnosed with cancer. Upon learning of this news, Ela instantly took emergency leave and was at home the same day. Within one year, Ela traveled to Kerala three times for about ten to fifteen days, using all the leave she could obtain.

John, by contrast, regretted that he could only return home after three years in Guyana because the journey took two or three days and the return flight ticket cost about USD 2,500, while the salary for nurses was not as high as in English-speaking countries. Because of this John was not informed of his father's accident. When he finally returned for a visit, John was shocked to notice the stiches in his father's shoulder. As his mother explained, "There's nothing he could do from so far away, so why bother him? He would only be tense. That's why I didn't tell him. He's not very near to us to come running to help." By avoiding talking about the father's accident, John's mother was protecting her son from what she deemed was unnecessary stress.

Being aware of the possibility of their parents' keeping health issues from them, some sons found a way around this, such as engaging a good friend to regularly drop by their parents' home with a smartphone or a tablet. In this way, a webcam made it possible for sons to check on their parents by looking for visual signs of ill health (see chapter 4). By contrast, daughters had less need for such arrangements; none of the parents I talked to ever mentioned they did "not want to bother" their daughters abroad by sharing their health-related concerns with them. John, too, mentioned that he would like to have a webcam connection with his parents more often to check on them and also to see them age. After three years away, it saddened him deeply to see how much their faces had changed, how they had aged while he was not aware of it. But he also realized that teaching his parents how to use a computer might be challenging.

Other circumstances, such as the COVID-19 pandemic, could also impact the ability to return home. When Aaron's father, already vulnerable because of his COPD, contracted COVID-19 in the spring of 2021, Aaron knew he could not fly home. His previous endeavor in traveling during the pandemic had entailed twenty-eight days of home quarantine in Kerala and then a repartition flight to return to his work in the United Kingdom. This experience had made it clear to him that an impromptu visit was not an option.

"I couldn't travel because there were no flights operating at that time. It was a very hard time; I couldn't do anything. I was absolutely stunned because I couldn't even go and see what was happening at home. Then, to return to the U.K. I would have to hotel quarantine for two weeks, which would cost around 2,000 pounds [USD 2,600], in a London hotel, very expensive. No." Aaron laughed at the thought of it. "Just no."

"How did you learn that your father was infected with COVID-19?" I asked.

I contact my parents every day, and one day in May 2021 my father was shivering and behaving very erratically, so I realized that something was wrong. I didn't waste any time. I told my mom, he must go to the hospital. It can be catastrophic if he doesn't get proper treatment! I googled for a private ambulance, which I first had to pay. Then they picked up my father, along with my mom, and they were taken straight to the hospital.

My father was admitted for five or six hours. They did some laboratory investigations of blood, and then they said he needed an ICU [intensive care unit] bed, but they also claimed that there weren't enough beds available. I had to threaten them by saying that I will contact the human rights council! I immediately started sending emails to the hospital management to complain, and I then also asked one of my friends who is a member of a local political party to call the hospital and talk to them. And that's what he did. The hospital management again asked for money, they wanted 50,000 Indian rupees [650 U.S. dollars] immediately. Finally, when I assured them that they would receive the payment, my father was admitted for fourteen days.

During that time, my mom was calling me all the time, every ten minutes, even during my work time. So I couldn't concentrate on my work, and I had to take a week of leave. After one week or so, my uncle started helping her, so things were better. But initially I was constantly on the phone. I took annual leave, not unpaid leave. I needed money, of course, and at the same time, I was absolutely stressed out. I was constantly on the phone, but at least in this way I was there for my mother, on the phone.

My mom and I always talk through a video call on WhatsApp. She's illiterate and doesn't speak English, but I taught her to use WhatsApp before I left to the UK, and she's completely comfortable with it. So my mom could see me, and I explained to her, go left, go right, speak to that person, fill out this form.

Aaron's narrative indicated that in the event of a health emergency, the frequency of calling home increased immediately and intensely. In fact, Aaron's presence at a distance in Kerala, through video calls, was so intense that he needed to take a week of leave from work. Frequent webcam interactions with his mother over the smartphone disturbed Aaron's attention and focus on his immediate physical environment. This negatively affected his concentration at work, to the degree that he was afraid of committing some serious professional mistake. The transnational care collective may not always be explicitly notice-able or perceived as something tangible, but its existence and impact could become palpable through the effort and concentration it required in times of health emergencies, such as this one. The engagement within the collective on those occasions could have concrete and critical consequences for members of the collective and people beyond them.

The smartphone was a key actor in supporting Aaron's organization of emer-gency care in Kerala for his father from the United Kingdom, from searching for a private ambulance—"Google is my friend," he told me with a laugh—to involv-ing various health care staff in the collective, directing his mother through the challenging health-care system, and speaking through video calls to the emer-gency doctor:

> I was speaking to people other than my mom over her phone, too, so phone was like a mediator for me. I told her to give her phone to my father's doctor, but he was very scared to take the phone from my mom, he said he might get the virus through it. I said all right, listen to my voice then. And so my mom held the phone with the webcam turned toward the doctor, and I was speaking with him at a distance.

At that time, the COVID-19 transmission pathways were not yet well under-stood, so the doctor was careful about handling material surfaces that had been in contact with another person. The image of Aaron talking to the doctor through a video call on his mother's phone—while keeping a physical distance from the doctor not to infect him with COVID-19—is especially striking as an example of the smartphone supporting caring co-presence at a distance, with the phone almost becoming a proxy for the physical body of a person. In this practice, the smartphone helped to enact three kinds of care simultaneously: health care for Aaron's father; care for Aaron's mother, who—as an older woman—struggled with establishing authority with the health-care staff in the hospital; and care for Aaron, who was deeply concerned about the situation. Within a single practice, care was thus distributed to several members of the transnational care collective at once.

Aaron's example further illustrates that digital technologies were not the only necessary nonhuman member when enacting health care at a distance. Money played just as important a role in supporting both chronic illness and emer-gency health events. One important reason for parents to have children abroad was as a sort of health insurance for their own old age because the children would provide the finances for health care expenses. Some writers on aging in India have expressed doubts about how many among the migrating children actually send remittances to their families (e.g., Falkingham et al. 2017; Sebastian 2020). However, various reports show that the households in Kerala that receive international remittances spend significantly more on health care and are also almost 50 percent more likely to seek health care from private providers than households without remittances (Khan and Chinnakkannu 2020). Additionally, households with family members in non-Gulf countries spend more on health care than those with family members in the Gulf countries (Sunny, Parida, and Azurudeen 2020). In 2007–2008, the estimated monthly international remittances in Kerala were about INR 67,000 (USD 870) per household, covering for almost half of the household's total expenditure, and almost 40 percent of those remittances were used for health-care costs (Mahapatro et al. 2015).

Monthly expenditures on health care, of course, fluctuate, depending on chronic illnesses that family members may have, so such expenses can rise sharply in times of acute health issues. Aaron regularly spent money on the supportive equipment to treat his father's COPD. Next to that, when his father became sick with COVID-19, Aaron took a personal loan from his employer in the United Kingdom to cover the unexpected hospitalization costs of INR 400,000 (USD 5,200). "That was a huge amount," he told me during a video call while he was buying a juice for himself in a shopping mall. "But I don't mind because it was for my father."

Another nurse told me, "Money is the basic thing that everybody wants, sure; there needs to be someone nearby to help with practical issues of health care, but for that money is also needed." Aaron's narrative is certainly in line with that. A nurse working in India could hardly afford the amount of money Aaron had to pay for a private ambulance and then an ICU bed for his COVID-19–infected father. In this way, the money provided by nurses abroad, either from their pay or even via short-term loans, was key to enacting health care at a distance.

IMAGES MIXING FEELINGS

One stiflingly hot afternoon in Kottayam, when I was leaving the English language class with a group of young students, I suddenly caught a glimpse of a photo on a smartphone that one of them, Yuti, was showing to a group of her classmates. From the stair above her, I could see that it was a photo of somebody's leg, and Yuti was showing it to the other young women, all nurses, and some were commenting loudly on what they saw. I hurried after them and asked Yuti what the photo was about.

"My aunt had an operation on her leg," she responded, stopping in the middle of the flight of stairs and thereby causing a traffic jam of bodies rushing toward the school exit. "I took some photos of it when I visited her in the hospital with my mom."

Yuti intended to send these photos further to her cousin, the aunt's daughter, who worked as a nurse in Italy and was not able to be by her mother's side at the time of the operation. It was a stressful time for both the mother and the daughter; they had waited for the operation for several weeks, and Yuti's aunt was very concerned about who would take care of her after the operation. Yuti's mother—her sister—was essential in calming her down and assuring her that she still had family nearby. But the main purpose of taking photos of the wound was to inform Yuti's cousin about the process: she wanted to see what had been done during the operation and how the wound was healing.

In transnational care collectives, family members commonly engaged in the practice of exchanging photos for the purpose of monitoring health. Sitting on his sofa in Australia, Anthony told me during our Skype conversation about how he used photos taken on a smartphone during his father's hospitalization.

ANTHONY: Two years ago my father was not so well; he had an ulcer in his foot, he needed help to walk, and he was also hospitalized for a long time. At that time, I received some photographs of the father's wounds. My brother took them because he had a good phone. So when he was visiting our father in the hospital, I asked him to take some photos. I'm a nurse, and I know how to assist the wounds, so I wanted to see what was happening: before and after surgery, what change did they make, how did the wound look, was it looking healthy, was it healing. . . . I didn't want to just rely on what the doctors say, I wanted to see by myself. Because I would have done that if I was present there in person, too. So I just wanted to do the same while away. I didn't ask for photos every day, but still, it helped.

T. A.: And did you give them some advice, or did you tell them to talk to the doctors or ask the doctors something?

ANTHONY: No, I didn't speak to the doctor, and I didn't give any advice, because the doctor informed them well, and they themselves have an idea of how to take care of themselves. My mother is a veterinary doctor, and my father is a well-informed person too. So I knew that they are quite independent.

Suddenly our conversation was disrupted by a siren, coming from Anthony's side. It became very loud, making it impossible to speak, so we stared at the screen silently for a few moments. "But I appreciated having the photos," Anthony continued once noise subsided. "With a picture, I had a better idea than just speaking over the phone."

The photos in Anthony's and Mary's stories were not taken specifically for the nurses abroad to provide any professional advice to their family members. Rather, the nurses required the photos so they would be informed of the situation as best as possible, to remain involved from afar by expressing their interest in this way, and to allay their own worries about their parent's health condition. As Anthony said, he would look at the wound if he were there in person, too, without the intention of doing anything particular about it. It was sufficient to be interested in seeing the photos, without necessarily acting on what they showed, at least so long as the healing seemed to progress well. In Winance's words (2010), paying attention is care.

Images, however, may be highly emotionally charged, and this makes certain photos more challenging to look at than others. While talking on the video call on WhatsApp, Aaron sent me a photo of his father two days after having been discharged from the hospital. I noticed that the photo was a screenshot of his post on Facebook. Aaron's father, a thin but youthful-looking man in a golden lungi and white shawl over his shoulders and arms, held his hands in front of his bare chest in a prayer position. It seemed he was expressing his gratitude, just as Aaron was in the long message he had written below the photo—thanking everyone for the thoughts and prayers that the family had received in their trying times.

"I put the news of my father's illness on my Facebook profile, just to ask people to pray for him. And yes, many people responded! See, if you have ten people praying for something, this automatically shifts energies, lifts the frequencies of the world. The power of the prayer is strong, immensely strong, as any ritual in this world, and that's the foundation of Christianity. The prayer has its own power; that's why I asked people to pray for my father."

For Aaron, receiving this photo of his father had given him a feeling of relief, and he gladly shared it with his contacts on Facebook and also with me. This illuminated another subtle care practice, prayer, which I mention in chapter 5. There, priests and close family members were asked to join in prayer for and with the sick person, but in Aaron's case social media amplified the power of the prayer by inviting his wider social network to participate. The photo of Aaron's father at home was shared as a way to celebrate his healing and thank those on Aaron's social media list who had engaged with Aaron's plea to pray, or at the very least they had hit the "like" button under his post to indicate their support.

Before his father returned home, Aaron's mother had sent him other, less hopeful images of his father lying in the ICU bed, hooked to all sorts of tubes and monitors. Those photos were much harder for Aaron to process. Even at the time of our conversation, almost a year after the event, Aaron still became emotional just thinking about them. Without me even asking, he said firmly that he would not share those images with me. "Frankly, those photos were very disturbing. Even after he was out of the worst, I was troubled by looking at them. It's sad to see someone you love in pain. At one point, I could look at them and analyze how bad he was in the first stage of infection. Eventually, I accepted that this is a part of life, and it got easier."

Many of my interlocutors believed that live images, streamed through the webcam, are superior to photographs because they afford interaction in real time. One person asserted that seeing a loved family member over a webcam was "better, of course" than talking on the phone with them because it made them "happier" to see the other person and to "feel as if you are there with them, in the same room." But I found that the webcam, too, could be emotionally disturbing. This was the case for Samuel and Raahel, Viju and Deepak's parents.

Viju and Deepak were brothers in their late 20s who had both migrated to the United Kingdom. Viju found work in a nursing home for people with dementia, while Deepak worked in a supermarket; they had been away for six and seven years, respectively. During this time, Deepak had married and had a son, who was a toddler at the time of our meeting. One of the first things I noticed when I entered the small jewelry shop that Deepak's parents owned was an iPad. It was placed on the glass display table, right next to Raahel who sat behind the counter, illuminated by the glow of golden necklaces, earrings, and bracelets around her. The iPad was proudly displaying a photo of a young child, Deepak's son, who was not even two years old. The boy had been born in London, and it took seven months before Deepak and his wife were able to travel to Kerala to stay there again for good (or at least that was what Raahel and Samuel were hoping).

While they eagerly had waited for the moment they would meet their grandson in person, Raahel and Samuel could see him on Skype. They had not owned a computer or smartphone, so they mostly had communicated with their sons by phone. But after he became a father, Deepak called his friend who owned the shop next-door to his parents. He asked him to visit his parents and call him by Skype (see chapter 4). Showing me a photo of their grandson—a boy with round cheeks and curly dark hair, reminding of a Renaissance angel—on their tablet, Deepak's parents recounted their experience of becoming grandparents at a distance:

SAMUEL: It was a dream come true. It was a mixed feeling to see him on Skype.
RAAHEL: We were excited. When we heard the sound of the baby, we were missing him. We couldn't hold him or touch him. The feeling was unbearable and difficult to explain. When they reached the airport in Kerala, with the baby, we were eager to see the baby's face. When I carried him, I was crying a lot. Our daughter-in-law gave the baby to Samuel. Everybody was crying. No one knew exactly what to do. He looked exactly like Deepak when he was a baby. It was very difficult to stay without seeing our grandson daily. We celebrated his first birthday in a grand way, we invited everybody around to the party. It was the happiest moment of our life.

For Raahel and Samuel, seeing their grandson on the webcam before they were able to hold him in their arms produced an "unbearable" mixture of feelings including happiness, excitement, and anguish. The webcam thus produced a new kind of feeling for which my interlocutors had no word thus far—it was simply "unbearable." The webcam had made the new grandparents intensely aware of the geographic distance between them and their grandson, and they felt there was nothing they could do about it.

Similarly, in Oman, Sara described her preference for photos over live video calls to communicate with her children, then teenagers, across the Arabian Sea. "I don't like Skype, actually. Seeing my children's faces on the webcam is just too hard for me. When I see them, I often start crying, and then they cry, and in the end everybody is just crying." Sara laughed, trying to mask her emotions.

In a way, the webcam has been too successful in its aim to make people feel almost as though they are together; but then they then must cope with the reality that they are not physically together. They can see and hear but not hold each other. While digital technologies afford various kinds of co-presence at a distance (Baldassar, Nedelcu, and Wilding 2016), the fundamental difference between being together through the webcam and being together in the same room remains—these two kinds of co-presence may be similar, even almost the same, but they are never entirely the same. While making them feel as if they are together, the webcam makes family members acutely aware of their physical separation, of the fact that the distance between them is considerable, and that the situation is not going to change any time soon. In other words, they become intensely aware of the vastness of the sacrifices they are all making.

AFFECTED BY DEMENTIA

On a sunny, stifling afternoon, an Ayurvedic doctor ushered me into a scantily furnished examining room of his clinic in central Kerala to introduce me to a potential research participant. There, a small, stout woman sat on a chair. Her name was Mercy. She was wearing a *salwar kameez*, a typical gown for a woman of her standing, senior and married with children. I tried to dissolve the uneasiness of our impromptu meeting by smiling a lot as I explained my study. Finally, she invited me to visit her home. She would cook dinner, she said, and I could meet her mother. I enthusiastically accepted.

When I entered Mercy's house, I immediately noticed her mother, sitting on the couch with a blank expression on her face. A woman in her 80s, she was afflicted with severe dementia, diabetes, and heart problems. She greeted me but did not seem interested in starting a conversation. Mercy led me into the kitchen, where she shared her mother's story while steaming rice and fried vegetables in the pan. In another pan, she had already fried some fish, and the sharp smell of it lingered in the air, slowly wafting through the open window that overlooked the back garden.

Despite having five children, Mercy's widowed mother found herself placeless in her old age. A general expectation was that one of her three sons would take her into his home where his wife would cook for, feed, and bathe her. Yet this was impossible in Mercy's mother's case: one son had cut all contact with her due to inheritance conflicts, the second son lived in another Indian state, and the third son had moved to Europe. Mercy's mother had spent her whole life in Kerala and did not want to relocate. Mercy herself was based in the United States, so her mother had had little choice but to move in with her other married daughter, Rosa, who lived not far from the family's ancestral home. But this arrangement was in contradiction with the common social conventions—in India, parents were not supposed to stay with their daughters, and Rosa's husband brought this up day in and day out (see chapter 5). Rosa, too, increasingly complained of the exhaustion of having to take care of a mother suffering from progressive cognitive decline. The brother in Europe had offered financial help, but Rosa brushed his offer aside. "Our mother needs somebody to feed her, by spoon, daily, and no amount of money could do that," Rosa reportedly told Mercy.

From the United States, Mercy used to call her mother regularly, but this was becoming increasingly difficult: how to talk on the phone with someone who had dementia and could not even remember she had a daughter, let alone one who lived abroad? Mercy still called, but she ended up mostly talking to Rosa about their mother's condition. She had also taken their mother into her own house while visiting Kerala for a couple of months that winter. In this way, she was providing care not only for her mother but also for Rosa by offering her some respite from the caring tasks, if only for a short time.

But keeping their mother at home, whether at Mercy's or Rosa's, was not a long-term solution. It simply couldn't be sustained. The two daughters did not have the knowledge or skills, but especially the patience, to take care of somebody with dementia, Mercy asserted. As a nurse, Mercy was familiar with specialized care facilities, and she approved of how older people were treated there. "People are in a group, and the carers teach them how to sit, eat, what to do. . . . It's good for them!" she said. "The nurses in these homes are trained properly, and they are paid for it so they should pay full attention to these people."

Mercy suggested to her siblings that they move their mother into a nursing home. And their reaction? They were strictly against it, as Mercy reported. "They said, people would ask, how can this be, there are five children, and no one can take care of her?!"

It had to do with dignity, with them being good children, with their whole family being a good family. In Kerala, and in India more generally as I described in chapter 3, old age homes were thought of as being full of the most devastated, poor people, people who came from bad families troubled by disagreements that led to bruised, if not broken, relationships. From our conversation, it slowly emerged that Mercy and her siblings indeed had a troubled relationship with their mother, with bitter memories that reached far back into their childhood. It seemed that placing their mother at an old age home would bring these intimate tensions to the surface and make them visible to everyone around them.

The disagreement over the nursing home remained a painful point for the siblings. Mercy was refusing Rosa's and her brothers' calls because she was so angry with them for not agreeing with her suggestion regarding a nursing home. She even declined their invitations to dinner out of fear of not being able to hide her feelings of frustration over the issue. Despite her siblings' protests, Mercy planned to visit a local nursing home. "But it's not only for my mother," she said. "I want to see it for myself, too." Her own plans for the future were uncertain. What would happen to her once her husband, many years her senior, passed away? She did not want to be a burden on either of her two daughters who were creating their own lives abroad. And yet, clearing the dishes from the table after dinner, Mercy said quietly, "Maybe, hopefully, one of my daughters will take me in."

Trying to understand the transnational care collective in Mercy's family was elusive. There were cracks in their collective, created by the onset of dementia, but also by decades of family conflict. The cracks appeared as the siblings' inability, unwillingness, or refusal to participate in the transnational care collective. What kind of collective can be formed, if at all, when some family members are unable to join it, or decline to participate, or are not allowed by other relatives to do so? Mercy could not care for her mother directly, if remotely, because dementia had made it impossible for them to have a conversation on the phone. Mercy's brother was denied participation because Rosa refused the remittances that he wanted to provide in an act of care. Another brother had declined to participate due to old disagreements.

Yet, as Annelieke Driessen (2018) suggests in her work on caring for people with dementia, the possibilities to participate in care are not necessarily a zero-sum game. In Mercy's family, care was indeed enacted, even though imperfectly and with limitations. Mercy may have thought that the care she and her siblings were providing was not good enough, but was this not care nonetheless? Although fraught with tension, ambivalence, and complex emotions, care was enacted through Mercy calling Rosa on a daily basis to follow their mother's state. Care was enacted through Rosa regularly negotiating with her husband about her mother living with them. Care was enacted through declining dinner invitations and through refusing phone calls out of frustration over differing views about the meaning and practices of good care for their mother with dementia. Care included Mercy's visiting nursing homes, even as these visits were accompanied by a lingering fear of her own imminent aging. Enacted in many different ways, care was neither easy on people's emotions nor effortless in terms of energy and time invested into finding solutions for an aging parent.

It seems, after all, that even a serious condition like dementia does not entirely preclude people and technologies from practicing care at a distance. Rather, declining mental and physical health shapes the participation in the transnational care collective in its own specific ways. Instead of connecting Mercy and her mother, the phone connected Mercy with Rosa in their joint endeavor to organize and discuss care for their mother. Dementia also shaped the relationship between Mercy and her brothers, who responded to the situation by offering money or declining to be involved.

As a degenerative condition that erodes capability in unpredictable ways, dementia is not as tangible as people or technologies, but it nonetheless importantly influences relations within families and how care may be done. Dementia—itself a condition that may be enacted in multiple ways (Mol 2002)—thus joined the transnational care collective as a participant of its own.

COVID CHILDREN

The COVID-19 pandemic, which took over the world in 2020, was the most devastating for older adults, both directly in terms of severe morbidity and mortality and indirectly through factors including isolation and income insecurity (HelpAge International 2021). Yet, as I was surprised to learn during my follow-up conversations, the nurses I spoke to—living in Australia, Germany, and the United Kingdom—were not exceedingly worried about their aging parents. In Kerala, they reasoned, houses are well spread out, and their parents would not socialize a lot anyway. One important social activity, going to church functions, was canceled anyway; clergy, who had often preached against technologies such as smartphones, suddenly embraced them and started transmitting mass online.[4]

"My mother is a housewife, so she doesn't go outside of the house much," Feni said in one of the voice messages that we exchanged over WhatsApp one Saturday in the summer of 2021. "My father mostly suffered because he had to stay at home for a while. He felt as if he were in a prison," Feni laughed. "He always complained that he wasn't allowed to go out and how annoying that was for him. So he regularly found an excuse to leave the house, to buy something important, like some medicines, just to go out a bit."

Despite their aging parents being in the most vulnerable demographic group during the pandemic, the everyday care within transnational care collectives became oriented toward children and even grandchildren. In this matter, the children's profession was significant: they worked in hospitals, a highly risky environment. Parents were reportedly much more worried than usual about their children's health, and they repeatedly reminded them to be careful, wear masks, and pay attention to patients potentially sick with COVID-19. The nurses I spoke with did not work on COVID-19 wards, so they felt relatively safe. Pia, however, caught COVID-19 soon after she moved to Germany in the midst of the pandemic. Luckily, her symptoms were mild, and she used home remedies to treat herself. But during the time of her illness, the dynamic in their family collective shifted; instead of her calling home daily, Pia's parents called her multiple times a day, and her mother advised her on which Ayurvedic treatments she should look for in her new country.

The COVID-19 pandemic further compromised the relationship between grandparents in Kerala and their grandchildren abroad due to the impossibility of returning to India during their longer holiday breaks, such as at the end of the calendar year. This was especially problematic for the nurses living in Australia and New Zealand who were under strict restrictions. Among them was Anthony and his wife, both nurses, who had not visited their families in Kerala since the end of 2019 until the time we talked in late 2021. They were pessimistic about being able to travel there any time soon, expecting the travel restrictions to continue for at least another year. In this situation, reliance on digital technologies to maintain their family relations transnationally had never been greater or more intense. As Anthony explained,

My mom and my grandmother would really like to spend some time with my daughter. It's such a sweet age when they are two, three years old. They are really missing that time. This is also when the little ones are starting to form their memories and develop their language. My daughter speaks a few words, sentences of Malayalam, but not more than that. We speak Malayalam at home, but my daughter watches a lot of TV, Netflix, she's probably learning words from there. She knows and understands everything that we say, she's kind of speaking a mix of English and Malayalam. She doesn't play with other Malayalam-speaking children since other children in her kindergarten speak English. She doesn't have a lot of friends of the same age from the Malayalam-speaking community.

Especially in the last year, because of the COVID-19 restrictions, families have not been mingling much. I think all this has affected children's language development. I read about "COVID children" recently, children who have problems with their language development because they aren't speaking or seeing many people, and yes, I'm concerned. I think it's very helpful for my daughter's speech development that my mom calls every day, sometimes twice a day.

She speaks with my daughter for at least twenty to thirty minutes on WhatsApp, on the webcam, so they know each other quite well. They speak a few words, often my daughter likes to dance when she's on the phone. She doesn't really speak much on the phone, but she's very happy to see that my mom is calling. She says hello initially, and then she moves on with her dance. She's pretty excited about these calls.

In Anthony's family, the dynamic of the transnational care collective shifted toward the granddaughter who was considered the most disadvantaged by the pandemic circumstances. Because her parents could not take her to Kerala, she was deprived of developing language skills in Malayalam, which in the future could endanger her relationship with her grandparents as their ability to communicate would decrease. In chapter 4, I write that in most collectives the children abroad call their parents, but the COVID-19 pandemic changed this pattern, at least for those with small children.

Anthony's mother took the initiative to call her granddaughter daily on Anthony's or his wife's phone. In this collective, video calls, video recordings, and photos became the primary modes of communication because they best supported the interaction between the granddaughter and her grandmother. Instead of language, they relied on nonverbal communication such as dance and play. So when transnational care collectives are extended to include grandchildren, especially babies and toddlers who are not yet able to speak, image-based digital technologies come to dominate within the transnational care collective (see chapter 4). As Anthony added,

> I send photos of my daughter, almost every day, to my mother through WhatsApp. If I get a good photo, or video record a dance, or she sings a song, I send it. Similarly, my mom would send images. Last week she recoded a baby goat she now has, and my daughter really liked it. It's all through WhatsApp, I don't use email or Facebook. Even though my mom is highly educated, she is not using emails, Skype, or other apps as they come along. But WhatsApp is quite user friendly, and she knows how to use it. When I spoke to you six years ago, my parents were not comfortable handling video calls, [and] Skype took some effort to master. But since then, smartphone has become quite popular, everyone has it, and most people have become comfortable with applications like WhatsApp.

The strong wish to interact with grandchildren was the greatest motivator for many older adults, especially grandmothers to learn new digital skills, including navigating social media. At the beginning of my fieldwork, I met several older women who attended computer classes at a local college specifically for this purpose. One of them, a widow in her 70s, told me about her struggle to overcome stigmatization as an older person and a woman. With anger still in her voice, she said, "I asked for the internet to be installed in my house, and the men told me, 'You're an old woman, what do you need the Internet for? You don't know what to do with it!'" But she insisted, and eventually succeeded.

Afterward, she faced similar problems of disinterest and dismissal due to her age and gender when she was looking for someone to teach her how to use the computer. Yet her strong wish to be in touch with her grandchildren in the United States—and specifically to see their pictures and video recordings regularly—motivated her to fight the prejudice. When I visited her at her home, she proudly and skillfully showed me the photos of her grandchildren on her iPad. "My son set up this cloud, and now I can see them whenever I want! It's nice because I don't want to disturb their daily life by calling. But these pictures are always there for me to see."

Stories like hers illuminate the gender and age discrimination in relation to digital technologies and further underline the importance of affect in digital empowerment. For older adults, and women especially, the greatest motivation to own digital devices and gain the knowledge on how to use them stemmed from emotions—the love and longing to be close to their grandchildren while geographically apart. Affect, then, was the fuel that stimulated older people to create transnational care collectives by ensuring that the necessary technological infrastructure was in place and then by gaining the needed skills to use digital technologies, despite the obstacles such as stigmatization that might be in their way.

THE FINAL IMPASSE

In March 2015, Manesh and I drove to Achamma and Pathrose's home for a follow-up visit. We had not brought any sweets or cakes, which would have been appropriate for a visit, but Manesh brought his blood pressure measuring device from his van, which he later described as "a very good idea"—it was his way of "giving something back to the people" rather than simply collecting research information from them. Achamma welcomed us and seemed pleased that we dropped by. We first sat on the veranda, but then she invited us into the sitting area in the house where Pathrose was also sitting. She sat next to him, suddenly looking tired. Her old sari was stained and bursting at the seams. Still, she seemed to be in good spirits. I noticed that the place was not as tidy as I was used to when visiting older people's homes. By way of explaining the state of the house, Achamma said that they used to have a maid, but she had left because she had some health problems of her own. They were not thinking of hiring another maid because it was too exhausting to even look for an agreeable person.

Some minutes after we sat down, Pathrose remarked that we were all playing in a movie, to which Achamma smiled, waved her hand, and said that he was "dreaming." She then shared with us that they had stayed with their daughter for about four months, but Achamma kept visiting their own house just to keep it clean. Then one day when she was returning from there, she tripped over a log, fell, and broke her arm. She said nothing to her family until the next day when her arm was obviously swollen. She had almost recovered now, and they had returned to their home several weeks earlier.

Achamma wanted to give lunch to Pathrose, and she told him to move from the chair to the kitchen table. "He needs to move a bit, keep active!" she said to Manesh and me. But Pathrose was resisting, and he told Achamma to bring lunch to him. Just as stubbornly, she refused, repeating that he should go and sit at the kitchen table. In the middle of our conversation, Achamma suddenly decided to take him there herself. It seemed very difficult for her to make him stand, even though she used the "walker," a Zimmer frame to support him. Pathrose stood up with much difficulty, so I asked Manesh if I should go and help them. At first, he nodded no, then changed to yes.

I held Pathrose on one side, and Achamma took his other hand. When we got through the door toward the dining room, she pulled him gently along, and I felt that he had trouble following; if she failed to pull, he would just stand at one spot for a long time before making a single step. Once in the dining room, I noticed the table and most of the chairs had been pushed against the wall. There was a large chair for Pathrose to sit in and a covered plate on the table, waiting for him. Under the table, ants were collecting some pieces of food, perhaps dropped at breakfast. Achamma noticed them, too, and she picked up the food from the floor. We helped Pathrose sit in his chair at the table. Achamma took the cover off the plate and told him to eat the cold rice with vegetable curries and fish fry.

All through this, Manesh had been waiting in the visiting room, but he finally joined us. He and I then stood, watching Pathrose eat slowly, while Achamma was busy by the kitchen sink, cleaning the dishes. Pathrose took a piece from his plate and offered it to us, saying, "Fish, have fish." Manesh politely declined.

At that moment, Achamma joined us with strawberry juice, not very strong, but still tasteful, for us. Manesh translated her explanation for me, with a meaningful smile: "It's the juice that Teresa brought." Then Achamma also brought green bananas on a plate, presenting them proudly, with a smile to us. Manesh looked at me and said, "I will share one with you if you don't mind." And so we did.

Achamma mentioned that Teresa was on her way over from the United States for a visit. She should reach them in just a day or two, and they were waiting for her call to know when exactly she would arrive. It was an eighteen-hour flight from California, and it took longer through Singapore than through Europe, Achamma added.

Pathrose finished his lunch, and Achamma tried to make him stand up again, but only to turn his chair toward the settee where Manesh and she then sat. Then she got out her mobile phone. She mentioned that she preferred talking on the landline, but it had been disconnected when they had moved to their daughter's house. Achamma found it difficult to type on the mobile phone, and the connection was not always good. But what was good about the mobile was that it was always there, even if there was power outage. Sitting down again, she used her left hand to look for Teresa's mobile number in the device. She was working very slowly on the phone, squinting her eyes, struggling to search through the phone menu. I asked if her accident had made it difficult to use the mobile phone; after all, she had broken her right arm. Shrugging her shoulders, she replied that she had learned to use her left hand. "What to do, you have to adjust."

Finally, Manesh stood up and went out to the veranda where he had left his blood pressure measuring device. He returned and measured the blood pressure for both of them; it was normal. When he was done, we said goodbye to Pathrose.

When I took his arm, he looked straight into my eyes with nothing but gentleness on his wrinkled face. Achamma followed us out to the gate and waved to us as we departed.

A few days later, I called the number that Achamma gave to Manesh, and Teresa answered the phone. I asked if it were possible for me to visit again, as this was a great opportunity to meet her in person. From her hesitant response, I understood that the time might not be appropriate. Not wanting to be intrusive, I let her think about my suggestion. I never heard from her again.

Confronting the end of life is never easy, and for transnational families such transitions were fraught with questions regarding what could and perhaps should be done better for all involved. Tensions arose among siblings, as in Mercy's case, on how to arrange good end-of-life care, or perhaps like in Teresa's case the parents were determined to live on their own despite having to cope with increasing difficulties. A central dilemma was whether children living abroad should return to Kerala and for how long, and parents' expectations differed according to whether the child in question was a son or a daughter.

For sons, parents could and sometimes would set a temporal limit on how long they agreed with them being abroad. John's mother, for example, told me, "It's ok for him to be away for ten years, so now he has seven more. He's a good son, he always helps us. But after ten years, he should come back home to us." John was a "good son" by providing financially for them, but perhaps in the future, his sister—who was also studying nursing—could take over the task of providing remittances while John would return home. John himself could foresee such a development of events in the future, but he also had an alternative plan, which was to move from Guyana, where he was working at the time of our meeting, to Canada. John could not imagine bringing his parents to Guyana, but Canada was a different story. There, he could obtain permanent residence for himself and eventually for his parents. Yet there also was much uncertainty in this plan: John's parents were not even aware of it, and perhaps they might not be willing to move across the ocean with him. Another risk was that the plan could fail altogether if John's visa was rejected, in which case he thought of returning to Kerala and finding a job near his ancestral home.

Among the female nurses, I only came across a single account of a nurse who had returned to Kerala to provide immediate care for a family member. Sara told me this story over a cup of coffee and a plate of dates when I visited her in Oman.

Years ago, my aunty was working as a nurse here in Oman, where she lived with my uncle. My father was working abroad as well while my grandparents lived alone in Kerala. Then my grandfather became sick and my aunty resigned from work. My uncle stayed here by himself. She left Oman in the spring, and the following year in winter my grandfather died. She cared for her father-in-law for less than a year. Everybody was talking about my aunty, what a good daughter-in-law she was to resign from her job and return to take care of her father-in-law. Very good she was!

Sara's eyes were wide with admiration as she described her aunt, and she kept nodding her head, although from her account it was not clear whether the aunt's decision to leave Oman was exclusively to care for her father-in-law or was there more to her decision. Still, this story from "years ago" was one of a kind; I recorded nothing similar involving recent generations.

Just as parents made no open claims on remittances from their daughters (see chapter 5), it was hard for them to make explicit claims for their daughters' physical presence. Daughters did, however, return home immediately for shorter visits of a few weeks or months—however much their work allowed—upon hearing news of their parents' declining health or even death. As I mentioned earlier, when Ela, who worked in UAE as a school nurse, heard that her mother had cancer, she took emergency leave right away and was in her natal home the very same day. In the year that followed she traveled to Kerala as frequently as her contract allowed her. When in UAE, Ela talked to her mother on the phone every day, just as she had done before the diagnosis. During some of those conversations, Ela would forget that her mother was sick, and she would continue talking without a break; but then her mother would not reply or would begin to breathe heavily, and only then Ela would remember. After her mother passed away, Ela returned to Kerala for the funeral: "It was most important for me to be there for the occasion. It was something I had to do, for her, but also for myself, to process the grief. I would find it impossible to do that from afar if I weren't able to travel."

Nevertheless, coming back to Kerala for good, and especially for the purpose of taking care of aging parents, was a difficult decision to make for anyone, daughter or son, so it happened very rarely. Deepak, who did return from the United Kingdom at his parents' request, said that it "felt as a sort of sacrifice" to relinquish the better employment and salary opportunities and generally the "higher quality of life" that he had had for six years. This dilemma reappeared as an important concern for the children abroad throughout my fieldwork.

In 2021, in my endeavor to better understand Syrian Christian ideas of good eldercare (see chapter 5), I came across Vasu, a priest who had lived in Italy for seven years before returning to Kerala when his wife became pregnant. In a video call via WhatsApp, he described his journey:

Our parents said they would like to spend time with their grandchild, so they asked us to return. It was more a request from my wife's parents because they had some health issues. I was hesitant to say no to them. Finally, I decided to return after I finished my PhD coursework. And here I am!

I have friends who still live abroad, caring for their parents in India by hiring maids for them. They tell me that I spoiled my future because I returned and declined an appealing job offer in Europe. I didn't refuse that offer because I'm rich, but because I decided to spend time with my family in India. In the end, it turned out that my decision was apt since my parents-in-law have passed away recently.

For some time, I was indeed doubtful about whether I made the right choice, but when they died, I felt that my decision was a good one. They were able to play with their grandchild, and they were happy. When we were abroad, we used to be in touch virtually, electronically, but the physical presence gave more peace of mind to them than the virtual relationship. They were a bit sick, my mother-in-law had kidney problems. It really brought her down that we were abroad. The presence of her granddaughter was very beneficial for her. She was able to spend almost three, four years with my daughter, and then last year both my wife's parents died.

For Vasu, the transnational care collective did not work efficiently enough to maintain it over time, especially as the aging and ailing parents-in-law felt that their time was slowly running out. The physical co-presence of their granddaughter even had a positive impact on Vasu' mother-in-law's physical health.

But then, our conversation turned toward the issue of finances, which was one of the main negative aspects of returning to Kerala, as Vasu explained:

Syrian Orthodox families in general don't have a lot of savings. We have land, we have properties, but we don't have a lot of cash in the bank. That is important for parents because in India the system is not like in Europe—European life is insurance life. I realized the beauty and effectivity of insurance when I was abroad, and then I got health insurance in Kerala, too.

In India, having health insurance is not so common among middle-class families, and when you go to the hospital most expenses are paid out-of-pocket.[5] So when my father-in-law started having heart issues, the doctor said that he needed an operation immediately, but we didn't have enough money for it. We arranged it, three or four months later, but it was too late. He died. So, finances have a major role in families.[6]

If I were in Italy at that time, I would earn enough to take a loan for the operation. The operation cost about 3,000–4,000 U.S. dollars, it was a bypass, an openheart operation. Yes, it's expensive here![7] My father-in-law was a high official in the police, a government servant, but his pension was not sufficient, and he didn't even pay attention to his health because he knew that he didn't have enough savings on his bank account to have an operation. So he hid the reality from us.

I still feel guilty about this—that I couldn't support our parents financially at the time when they needed it. If I had stayed abroad, I could have helped.

"This is a dilemma, isn't it?" I let Vasu catch a breath. "Do you come back home so your parents can spend time with their grandchildren, or do you stay abroad and provide them with money to cover for their health expenses?"

> Yes! See, if at least one of us were abroad, I or my wife, it would still be possible to provide enough money. But for me, that is another problem. I expect a family—husband, wife, and their children—to be always together. Otherwise, why should we get married? I believe in a life together because we just have one life. If I can't spend time with my daughter when she is young, when she needs a father, and then five or ten years later I come back and tell her "I love you" a hundred times—it doesn't make sense. So I preferred to have a family life rather than me staying abroad alone.

"What do you then think of those nurses who live abroad by themselves while their husbands and children are in Kerala?" I asked.

"It's an immense sacrifice. They are losing an important part of their life—spending time together with their children and their spouse—which is not happening for them, and they are never getting that time back."

In the context of low salaries and high health-care costs, how could adult children, especially those from the lower and middle classes, ensure good care for their parents? Inherent in this question is the ethics of decision-making. There are several options to choose from, each with its own plethora of consequences. None of them is perfect, yet one must be taken.

Vasu's response suggests several possibilities. The first one was to stay at home; in this way, the children could provide their parents with "peace of mind" and the joy of being near their grandchildren, with a positive influence on their grandparents' health. This option came with a caveat: the family might then not have enough money to pay for aging parents' health-care expenses, especially if the need appeared suddenly.

The second option was also an uneasy compromise: one spouse—in the case of my study, usually the wife-nurse—worked abroad while the other spouse and children remained in Kerala. In this way, the family had, presumably, enough money to cover even excess health-care expenses, and most of the family members lived close to each other or even shared their residence. Yet this arrangement came at great emotional expense of the separated nuclear family, especially for the adult child/parent who was living abroad alone.

To avoid such physical separation, many decided for the third option, which was for the whole nuclear family to leave Kerala and work abroad, generating a steady cash flow through which many family members could be sustained for years and their health care could be covered, from the costs of chronic illness to unexpected emergencies. This, of course, made it impossible to live together and share the small joys and struggles of life side by side. A possibility which Vasu did not mention was for the parents to move abroad to live with their children; however, as my fieldwork showed most parents did not favor this idea, citing irreconcilable differences of weather, friends, and food.

The third option on Vasu's list, while not without its tensions and ambivalences, remained the most common among nurses from Kerala. This was to migrate internationally with their own families and enact care through transnational care collectives. In the end, what mattered more than anything else were affective ties, however complex, fluid, and challenging, which were the genuine glue of caring across distance. In Aaron's words,

> The real relationship starts from the heart. If you have a heart to care about people around, obviously you have a good attachment. You see, I can get my parents' vibe very quickly. If my mom is crying, I can understand, I can feel it in my heart, because we're very close through the heart, through the feelings and emotions, not through the distance. Distance is just a number. And it's true, I can't run and visit them, but they're always inside my heart. I can sense them. They can sense me even. It's an attachment, it's an emotion that never fades. It's good that I have a phone and can contact them, with the help of world wide web. [Aaron laughs.] But yeah, indeed. [His voice softens.] I just miss them.

Transnational care collectives do not act as a perfect replacement of a life in physical proximity. That would be an impossible aim to reach because feeling "as if" in the same place through the phone or the webcam is never the same as actually being in the same place. A technologically mediated co-presence is not equal to physical co-presence; digital technologies influence how people relate to each other, in ways that I describe throughout this book. Nevertheless, although enacting care and health care more specifically through transnational care collectives may not be the perfect option, for many families it was and continues to be the optimal—and the most ethical—one.

CONCLUSION

A senior Indian woman, wearing a nighty with a floral print, is lying in her bed, staring with a despairing look past her nightstand where, next to a collection of bottles and sheets of pills, a smartphone is vibrating tirelessly. She takes a deep breath and finally forces herself to look at her phone. Four messages from Nurse Anita are waiting for her on WhatsApp. The next moment the woman is up on her feet, making her bed. When all the creases in the spotless white bed linen are smoothed out, she takes a photo. Her face becomes serious when she contemplates how to send it through, but then she manages rather quickly, and she is visibly relieved. Then she sits on a settee and listens with interest to all those audio messages that got her out of bed.

The messages have the power of the morning sun. The woman's face brightens as she opens the curtains, ready to take on another day. With her hair now neatly combed in a bun and wearing a sari the color of cherry blossoms, she opens her sketchbook and immerses herself in painting. Once done, she takes photos of her artwork with her smartphone and sends them away. But who is on the receiving end?

A young woman, "Nurse Anita" as the smartphone screen reveals, is hanging her laundry on a balcony, and she smiles at the familiar tone that her smartphone emits. Finally, the two women are joined in a video call, and seeing each other makes them smile. They end their conversation by sending each other kisses through the screen. The line "What brings you closer, is between you" appears on the screen to wrap the one-minute advertisement into a perfect bundle of warm-hearted emotions.

Released in July 2020, just months into the COVID-19 pandemic, the WhatsApp campaign #ItsBetweenYou was exceptional: while the major online platforms and social media platforms were producing campaigns that targeted young, well-situated professionals and families with school-going children (Cabalquinto and Ahlin 2021), WhatsApp created a short film that addressed older adults, and particularly women who lived alone. The connection between the two women in the ad remains implicit, but the most straightforward interpretation is that they are a daughter who is a nurse, living and working in some distant location, and her mother. The advertisement very likely hit close to home for many nurses and their parents in my study: digital technologies—and in recent years specifically WhatsApp—have become a "lifeline" and "a safe space" where people can share the most intimate details of their everyday lives (Srivastava 2020).

Because of the accessibility of digital technologies even to people from lower economic classes, "cheap calls" have been described in the academic literature on migration and transnational families as the "social glue" for those separated by geographic distance (Vertovec 2004; cf. Haenssgen 2019). In this book, I aimed to understand the precise influence of the digital technologies people use daily— often by the hour, by the minute—on them and their most intimate relationships, how these devices shape what care comes to mean when it is practiced at a distance, and how to do such care well. I have found the science and technology studies of care, specifically the material semiotic approach, to be helpful in providing the vocabulary and analytical tools to articulate a reply to these questions, as it is formulated in this book, for now. In a nutshell, this is the answer: when geographic distance is introduced among family members, people enact care with the help of digital technologies through transnational care collectives. What are these collectives, how are they established, and how do people practice care within them?

As global assemblages of people and digital technologies, transnational care collectives support the enactment of care through practices such as frequent calling, sharing everydayness by recounting minute details of daily life on the phone, and spending time together through webcams, sometimes in silence. Each transnational care collective has its own dynamic, as family members tinker with different kinds of technologies, telecommunication infrastructures, time zones, work and social schedules, and multiple kin and non-kin members who become included over time, with different intentions and levels of intensity. Tinkering is a task that is never fully completed; it demands considerable effort, especially in the first days, weeks, and months after a family member moves abroad. The dynamic of transnational care collectives is bound to change through time and space as migrating adult children move from one country to another and technologies evolve, but also when tough decisions must be made in the face of failing health or when other circumstances such as the COVID-19 pandemic intervene. Furthermore, the polymedia environments (Madianou and Miller 2012) within which families can pick and choose their digital technologies change with different national and natural contexts, as technologies develop and become increasingly user friendly, and as people's health becomes ever more delicate.

As a relatively recent phenomenon, transnational care is about finding one's way in an uncharted territory of what makes good care at a distance. Empirical ethics draw attention to how norms of care and filial obligations are not fixed but are fluid and subject to change. For the Syrian Christian families of migrating nurses from Kerala, frequent calling has become a new filial duty through which the children appease their parents' feelings or fears of abandonment. Importantly, however, calling as care is not just about communication. It involves very practical health interventions, too, such as giving advice on medicine, monitoring chronic illness, ordering an ambulance, and negotiating health-care access when the need arises. Through their different affordances, various types of technologies impact how people relate to each other in specific ways, either by inviting them to increase their verbal communication, as a phone does, or by enabling them to be comfortably silent together, as the webcam allows. Tinkering with technologies further includes being attentive to people's emotional responses. Indeed, the webcam affords seeing each other in real time, but this is not necessarily a better way of connecting: live video calls are almost too efficient in making people feel as if they were together while they are physically apart, and this can trigger painful emotions, described by my interlocutors as "unbearable feelings." Through visual images, a webcam may also reveal unpleasant information that people would prefer to keep secret in order to protect their loved ones from worry and concern.

Transnational care collectives do not stand on their own but are part of a broader ecology of care at a distance. This ecology is digitally shaped, and it further includes sociomaterial, economic, temporal, affective, religious, and even spiritual spheres. To start with, the establishing and maintaining of collectives is contingent on affective relations between family members—digital technologies do not initiate calls by themselves (for now, at least). There are other—affective—reasons that motivate people to pick up their phones and search for their mother's, father's, daughter's, or son's phone number and push the green button or swipe the green circle on the screen. Affective relationships, of course, transcend simplistic descriptions; they are complex, ever evolving, and include a plethora of emotions. The quality of people's relationships, both before migration and as they develop throughout years of living apart, shapes transnational care collectives in specific ways as it influences the level of participation of each family member in their collective. Feelings of love, attachment, and concern are the greatest motivator for aging parents to learn how to use new digital technologies, particularly when grandchildren are in question. This shows that the glue that keeps people connected across times and places is not "cheap calls" in and of themselves (Vertovec 2004) but rather the affective ties for which evolving digital technologies open and hold space.

Further, material semiotics make it possible to understand care as well as gender and kinship as things that are enacted and therefore flexible and subject to change through different situations and practices. Enactment, radical relationality, and empirical ethics (Mol 2002; Pols 2013, 2014) are the theoretical tools that illuminate how people form relations not only with other people, but also with technologies, and how these relations between humans and nonhumans in turn enact care as well as gender and kinship. This is a fundamentally different analytical approach from treating notions like care, gender, and kinship as analytical lenses through which ethnographic data are theorized (Harbers, Mol, and Stoll-meyer 2002; Hoogsteyns 2008).

In this book I have shown how these notions are enacted not only with the help of technologies but also with money in its various forms. In the Syrian Christian families I encountered, the idioms of suffering and sacrifice were mobilized as affective mechanisms to support and justify the continuous money flows that are a prerequisite for transnational care collectives and, together with digital technologies, contribute to maintaining these collectives over time. Remittances are particularly significant for aging parents because in India only a fraction of the population receives a pension and most health care expenses are paid out of pocket (Ahlin, Nichter, and Pillai 2016). As a parental investment in education and a return on this investment in the form of remittances, money participates in enacting international migration as a care practice rather than an act of elder abandonment.

On a practical level, the narratives presented in this book offer valuable lessons for the introduction and implementation of technologies in health care in forms such as telemedicine, telemonitoring, e-health, and digital wearable devices. After all, understanding what could be learned about everyday digital technologies that may serve to improve technologically supported health care was my initial inspiration for this research. The number of people included in my study was relatively small, as is often the case in ethnographic research. Rather than making generalizing claims, my intention was to explore in depth the intricate complexities at the nexus of care, technologies, aging, and migration. The findings from one case study—such as transnational families from Kerala—can be translated into other situations to find meaningful solutions.

My research, for example, shows that regardless of their age, people did not make much use of new, innovative, specialized technologies that were created specifically for the purpose of improving health or maintaining physical and mental abilities. Instead, what served them best for care was the most easily available, affordable, and accessible digital technologies that were initially designed for the most general purpose of communication. Surprisingly, however, within the transnational care collectives that these generic devices supported, a major goal of people's interaction was not communication in the sense of an exchange of information. Instead, the most important aim was enacting care through the many practices—some of which are quite implicit—that are brought to light in this book. The purpose of daily calling, for example, is not to share some trivial information. Rather, the goal of making calls consistently and frequently is a way to build and maintain trust, which is crucial for people to follow health-related advice when the need for it arises.

So instead of focusing exclusively on constant technological innovation, and then running into challenges deriving from digital inequalities, illiteracy, and interoperability, I suggest that the question should be how to make best use of general digital technologies for health, in ways that are not always obvious. Digital technologies are often already available and affordable to people at large, although admittedly they are less accessible to people who struggle with using digital technologies due to physical limitations. Involving older people in the technological design process would be a fruitful approach to develop, for instance, smartphones that are specifically made for people with poor sight or hearing or with Parkinson's disease (see also Prendergast and Garattini 2015). The uptake of digital and other technologies among older adults could be further stimulated by appropriate, clear user manuals, such as that developed by HelpAgeIndia (see chapter 2). Such manuals remain surprisingly rare, and so older people are most often dependent on others to help them with deciphering the working of digital technologies.

Basic digital literacy is essential to establishing transnational care collectives, and I found that younger family members who had the appropriate knowledge, especially in case of visual technologies, often played a key role. They could set up video calls and teach older adults how to use WhatsApp. In India, institutions such as HelpAge India (2020) have also been actively working on empowering senior citizens through their workshops on digital technology use. Such endeavors are highly valuable and especially efficient if they are guided by the awareness of what motivates older people most to engage with digital technologies. For example, in my research, older people were not greatly interested in technologies for the purpose of health, for example, by using various health-oriented apps. But they could be incredibly inspired by their wish to be connected to their family members across distance; this was particularly true for women who were grandmothers.

The notion of transnational care collectives also highlights the fact that technologies not only support care but also demand it for themselves. As this book argues, care within collectives becomes distributed among its human and nonhuman participants. Care in the form of regular maintenance—such as keeping the batteries charged and the credit full—is necessary work, which further requires financial resources to keep the collective functioning. Additionally, although some care practices, notably hands-on care, were not possible in transnational care collectives except through occasional visits, that did not mean that the care workload decreased for family members. People did not care less because they were far away; rather, they started caring differently. In a transnational context, digital technologies and money both shaped their emerging care practices.

Technologies, whether specialized for healthcare or common digital devices, thus do not necessarily and automatically decrease the workload and cost of care. Instead, they change the nature of work, the routines of care, the required skills, and the distribution of expenses (see also Pols 2012). This is yet another relevant finding for the health care industry and policy makers to take on board when considering the implementation of technologies in their operational processes. Technologies are often applied in health care to facilitate some tasks with the aim of achieving greater efficiency. But it is essential to evaluate, in each individual case, how these newly introduced devices and systems interfere with the established understandings and practices of care, claim care in the form of maintenance, and require additional skills and knowledge from those who engage with them. As this book demonstrates, ethnography is a particularly valuable method of examination of such cases since it makes it possible to explore the most implicit and unexpected impacts of technologies on people and their care practices within their broader sociopolitical contexts.

Additionally, digital technologies cannot be expected to entirely replace in-person interaction. Technologically mediated relationality is precisely that—it is mediated through technologies and therefore not exactly equal to non-mediated relationality. The webcam offers a particularly poignant example: this device is remarkably efficient in creating feelings of copresence at a distance, and at the same time it makes people acutely aware of the physical distance between them. Enacting care through transnational care collectives is often the preferred option when other options (such as living together or nearby) are impossible for the well-being of all involved. Yet for these collectives to function over time, regular visits in-person are essential. The families I met during my fieldwork emphasized the joy and importance of returning to Kerala once a year or more, if required, for example, by a health emergency. These visits were necessary for migrating children to nurture strong personal relations and trust with their parents, but also with their extended family members, friends, and neighbors who could then be included in transnational care collectives should the need arise. This indicates that care at a distance is significantly supported through hybrid rather than exclusively digital interaction, even if the temporal intervals between in-person contact are relatively long—a discovery that is highly pertinent to establishing systems of telemonitoring.

As I show throughout this book, material objects—in this case everyday digital technologies—need to be taken seriously as participants in human relations because they shape people's relations and even their very identities. They do so in subtle, yet decisive ways. The workings of everyday digital technologies might be difficult to discern because of their often seamless and complete integration into people's daily lives; in the words of Carla Risseeuw (1991; see Gamburd 2008, 23), "The fish don't talk about the water." However, not paying attention to what technologies co-enact together with people and what the consequences are may have important hidden costs: the practical and emotional labor of care at a distance may be unacknowledged or underappreciated, and even more, shifting people's identities, roles, and statuses may involve concealed abuses and misuses. As interaction via digital technologies is never exactly the same as in person, these devices may contribute not only to care but also to misunderstandings and conflict, which may oblige people to engage in constant work of reducing this risk. On the other hand, geographic distance may be an implicit but essential way for people to avoid interpersonal conflict or the overwhelming sense of responsibility or dependence (see also Madianou and Miller 2012).

Beyond influencing interpersonal relations in such paradoxical ways, engaging with digital technologies can include other harms. Take the WhatsApp advertisement, which opens this conclusion, as an example. The ad offers a glimpse into a well-oiled transnational care collective (or so one could assume): an aging mother, her daughter living somewhere far away, and their smartphones with a social media platform that suits them best at that moment. Among many other implications it carries, the ad also suggests that the information shared between the two women is safe to stay between them. However, it is worth remembering that "if the product is free, you're the product" (Doffman 2021). Digital technologies, including the social media that commonly participate in transnational care collectives, are created, maintained, and developed by technological corporations that work on business protocols. These operations, like national telecommunication infrastructures, are an "absent presence" (Law 2002), an element that is hidden from plain view yet fundamental to the functioning of technologies. When people engage with digital technologies due to need or convenience—including that of practicing care at a distance—they give away their most intimate data, often without being aware of it or any of the implications this could have. Such extracting of personal data for profit is at the core of data capitalism (Couldry and Mejias 2019). It is therefore important to be aware that we, individually and by accumulation collectively, decide what to make of the technologies that we create, which of them we engage with, and how often, for what purposes, and in what ways. The Responsible Today Initiative, which was launched in India in 2022, is a promising attempt to tackle such individual and societal challenges brought about by the intensified presence of digital technologies, and hopefully it is an example for many more to follow.[1]

Through exploring transnational care collectives of one particular group of people, notably the Syrian Christian families of migrating nurses from Kerala, this book offers insights that are valuable for the development and implementation of technologies in health care and that advance discussions of transnational care by doing "bridgework" among anthropology and science and technology studies (Rodríguez-Muñiz 2016). Most importantly, however, I hope that I have managed to bring to light how something as mundane as picking up a mobile phone to call a family member is actually an astonishing, complex practice of care. It is such because it matters so deeply to the people who do it. Just consider, for a moment, the last time you called your mother or your father or perhaps your children to ask them how they were doing and how their day was. After having read this book, I hope you will agree with me about just how significant it is that you called, and that they answered.

ACKNOWLEDGMENTS

This book would not have come to light without many people who have inspired and supported me, each coming my way exactly at the right moment. I'm grateful to all who were, directly or indirectly, involved in the making of this book and in my professional and personal growth. First, to all the people in and from Kerala who answered my calls, opened their doors to me, and welcomed me into their intimate lives: I am immensely thankful to you for sharing *dosha*, jackfruit, and your stories with me. I feel these pages barely do justice to the depths of your lived experiences, and I will continue to strive toward writing them better.

In Kerala, I was selflessly helped by many people who remain anonymous in these pages to protect their and our interlocutors' privacy. Among them, I am especially indebted to two splendid women, one who introduced me to Kerala and one who joined me on many of my travels through the state to visit families and sometimes also just for fun—you know who you are. I am deeply grateful to you for your practical assistance, including in some cases interpretation and transcription, and for your daily support, care, and friendship that goes far beyond this research.

Thanks also to my friends and colleagues in Kerala, Hari Kumar Bhaskar and Gopukrishnan Pillai, and to Sebastian Irudaya Rajan for hosting me in the Centre for Development Studies (CDS). Throughout the years, I have learned a great deal from the scholars who have worked in Kerala and elsewhere in India: Bianca Brijnath, Ester Gallo, Claudia Lang, Mark and Mimi Nichter, Marie Percot, Manja Bomhoff, Caroline Osella, Ira Raja, Harish Naraindas, and William Sax. I am particularly grateful to Sarah Lamb for her support and encouragement along the years; your generosity and kindness are a perpetual source of inspiration.

The main theoretical arguments in this book were developed during my doctoral studies at the University of Amsterdam (UvA). To my supervisor Jeannette Pols, thanks for taking care of both me and my writing. This book wouldn't have been what it is without your guidance, grounded in patience and trust. To Kasturi Sen, my co-supervisor at Wolfson College, University of Oxford, I am grateful for your selfless commitment and intellectual challenges, and for making sure that "the emotions are in."

At UvA, this book and I have benefited from the generosity of many. During my studies, Kristine Krause and Annelieke Driessen established and chaired the *Writing Care* seminar where many pages of this book were discussed, dissected, and reassembled. I'm indebted to these events and those who participated, including Shahana Siddiqui, Eva Vernooij, Carla Rodrigues, Laura Vermeulen, Sherria Ayuandini, Annekatrin Skeide, Christien Muusse, Ellen Algera, Ildikó Plájás, Sarita Jarmack, and Ariane d'Hoop. I am further grateful to Sjaak van der Geest,

Anita Hardon, Annemarie Mol, Annelies Moors, Amade M'Charek, Ria Reis, Emily Yates-Doerr, Else Vogel, and the late Mario Rutten for engaging with different parts of this work. In 2016, Eileen Moyer, Silke Hoppe, and I organized an ethnographic writing workshop that culminated in an unforgettable event which we called Ethnographic Slam. To my co-organizers and to Julie Livingston and Robert Desjarlais, who joined us as lecturers, thank you for making that workshop a reality and a dream.

This book benefited from many discussions at workshops, seminars, symposiums, and conferences around the world. To start with, I'm thankful to the members of the Philosophy of Care group at Amsterdam Medical Center, especially Dick Willems and Maartje Hoogsteyns. I'm grateful to Nelly Oudshoorn, Tamar Sharon, Laura Merla, and Anna Mann for their kind engagement with my early thoughts on transnational care collectives. Thanks to Kasturi Sen for arranging my presentations at the University of Oxford and to those who attended, particularly Marcus Banks and Matthew McCartney, for their comments. In 2016, Fangfang Li and I co-organized a panel on multisited and digital fieldwork at the Association of Social Anthropologists of the United Kingdom and the Commonwealth conference; thanks to the panel discussants Loretta Baldassar and Nicolescu Razvan, and to the panelists for their inspirational contributions on digital technologies and the field site.

Further, I'd like to express my gratitude to Daniel Miller, Megha Amrita, Jason Danely, Christiane Brosius, Roberta Mandoki, Annika Mayer, Brigit Obrist van Eeuwijk, Piet Van Eeuwijk, Jana Gerold, Urmila Goel, and Earvin Cabalquinto for inviting me to various panels and for thinking with me through care, aging, migration, and digital technologies in seminar rooms, during online sessions, and at dinner tables. Among the participants at these events, I have learned from conversations with Michele Gamburd, David Prendergast, Monika Palmberger, and Katrien Pype.

In 2015, I was honored to be invited to the Wenner-Gren workshop as a conference monitor; thanks to the workshop organizers Lenore Manderson, Mark Davis, and Chip Colwell and to the participants, especially Susan Erikson, Cristiana Giordano, Ravi Sundaram, and Junko Kitanaka, for discussing my early fieldwork findings among the hills of Sintra, Portugal. I'd like to thank Peter Simonič for an invitation to publish and present parts of this work at the University of Ljubljana, and to Gorazd Andrejč for invitations to discuss empirical ethics at the University of Groningen.

At the many American Anthropological Association annual meetings I attended throughout the years, I was lucky to encounter Danya Glabau, Nayantara Appleton, and Christy Spackman—thanks for your support and acknowledgment of my work, which came at a point when encouragement was much needed. Daisy Deomampo, Lynnette Arnold, Kristin Yarris, and Cati Coe, thank you for engaging with my work and offering feedback at those meetings. This

book also benefited from conference hall conversations I had with Jay Soko-
lovski, Janelle Taylor, Valerie Olson, and Philip Kao. Roberta Raffaetà, your
friendship has been invaluable to me ever since Montreal! Amy Dao, I'll always
appreciate our Book Writing Mastermind that got this project started on sheer
passion, and your comments on the early chapters were invaluable—thank you.
And Loretta Baldassar, the image of us, engrossed in discussion on material
semiotics in the middle of a Vancouver souvenir shop, with the Indian incense in
the air, remains imprinted in my memory.

Parts of this book were previously published in the following journal articles:
"Only Near Is Dear? Doing Elderly Care with Everyday ICTs in Indian Transnational Families," *Medical Anthropology Quarterly* 2018; 32 (1): 85–102; "Frequent
Callers: 'Good Care' with ICTs in Indian Transnational Families," *Medical
Anthropology* 2020; 39 (1): 69–82; "Shifting Duties: Enacting 'Good Daughters'
through Elder Care Practices in Transnational Families from Kerala, South
India" (co-authored with Kasturi Sen), *Gender, Place and Culture* 2020; 27 (10):
1395–1414; and "From Field Sites to Field Events: Creating the Field with Information and Communication Technologies (ICTs)" (co-authored with Fangfang
Li), *Medicine, Anthropology and Theory* 2019; 6 (2), no. 4931. Thanks to all the
involved peer reviewers and to the journal editors Vincanne Adams, Lenore
Manderson, Kanchana Ruwanpura, Eileen Moyer, and Vinh Kim-Nguyen, and
to special issue editors Narelle Warren and Dikaios Sakellariou, for their support
through the publishing process.

Most research for this book was funded by the European Commission through
the fellowship International Doctorate in Transdisciplinary Global Health
Solutions—Erasmus Mundus Joint Doctorate Trans Global Health Programme
and the Erasmus Mundus 2009–2013 Programme Guide, version 11/2013, Specific
Grant Agreement 2013–1479. This funding was extended by the Health, Care and
the Body Program group at the Department of Anthropology, Faculty of Social
and Behavioural Sciences, UvA. I am immensely thankful for this support.

This book would not be what it is without Lenore Manderson—my heartfelt
gratitude for accepting this work in the *Medical Anthropology* series and for reading every page with utmost care. I am deeply honored to have had you as my
year-long mentor and now editor. Thanks also to Kimberly Guinta at Rutgers
University Press for making the publishing process such a pleasant experience.

Beyond academia, thank you Miriam Tocino, Marija Marić, Patricia Junge,
Babette van der Zwaard, and Marieke van Atten for listening and offering support on so many occasions. Vesna Nikolić and Chris Boothe, thanks for keeping
my body and mind sane and sound through the years of research and writing.

Finally, my family proper. To my mother, *mati*, I'm deeply thankful for your
support, for instilling in me creativity as one of the greatest values, and for
encouraging me to follow my own path. It is you—and our close relationship
across distance—that is at the heart of this work. To Milan and Mojca, thank

you for providing me with the much-needed time and space to write through the years. *Hvala!* To Mitja, for sticking with me all along this adventure, for listening, and for your encouragement through the tricky times—you are my rock to lean on, and I'm forever grateful to have you by my side. And then, to Aria: I started writing this book after you were born, and it has grown along with you. Meanwhile, I have clearly been flying on love fuel. Thank you for coming into my life and for simply being you. I will always pick up your call.

APPENDIX
Note on Methodology

In finding relevant families to talk to about care through digital technologies, my main criterion was that the family had one or more children working abroad as a nurse, regardless of where the children lived and for how long they were abroad. I carried out interviews and participant observation among members of thirty-three such families, in most cases only with the adult children-nurses (sixteen), and in other cases with multiple family members (thirteen) or only with the parents or parents-in-law (four). Additionally, I interviewed five nurses who had worked abroad then retired and returned to Kerala permanently or for a few months each year. My data was enriched by several group interviews, conducted at the English language school, and brief chats and interactions with numerous other people I met throughout my fieldwork.

Besides visiting and interviewing, I stayed with four families for a while. I spent two days with one family in Kerala and between two and fourteen days with members of three families in Oman and United Arab Emirates. Throughout my fieldwork in India, I lived with two families who had no children abroad (one in northern and one in southern India), which enabled me to observe and learn about conventional eldercare practices.

In all families in my study, every adult used some digital devices, from landline phones or simple mobile phones, to smartphones, laptops, tablets, and personal computers. They had various levels of knowledge, skills, and abilities regarding digital technologies and used these devices accordingly.

All personal names, some names of places, and some personal details have been modified to ensure anonymity.

Overview of Study Participants (2014–2022)

Children and parents**

	Name	Age*	Gender	Religion	Country of residence	Family	Parents' occupation (source of income)	Field sites/events
1	Sara	40	Female	Christian—Orthodox Syrian	Oman	Father (70) and mother (64); husband and children in Kerala; one brother in U.S., one brother in U.K.	Small-scale farmers	Kerala, Oman
2	Usha	39	Female	Christian—Orthodox Syrian	Oman	Husband, two children in Oman; father (73) and mother (63), sister in Kerala; one sister in Kuwait, one sister and brother in Oman (all siblings nurses); mother-in-law in Kerala	Small-scale farmers	Kerala, Oman
3	Teresa	40	Female	Christian—Roman Catholic	U.S.	Mother, father; two sisters in Kerala, one sister nurse in Kuwait	Father retired office worker	Kerala, phone
4	Mary	24	Female	Syrian Christian—Kananaya	U.K. (planned), later in New Zealand	Father (63) and mother (58); two elder sisters nurses in U.K.	Father a driver, landowners	Kerala, Skype

Overview of Study Participants (*continued*)

	Name	Age*	Gender	Religion	Country of residence	Family	Parents' occupation (source of income)	Field sites/ events
5	Joy	27	Female	Christian—Orthodox Syrian	Saudi Arabia, Germany	Mother (50s), father (60s), younger brother in Kerala	Father electrician	Kerala
6	Teena	28	Female	Hindu	Maldives	Father and mother; sister married in Kerala	Father a worker on other's farmland	Kerala
7	John	32	Male	Christian—Orthodox Syrian	Guyana	Mother (50s), father (60s); recently married a nurse; sister studying nursing in another Indian state	Father a plumber, small-scale farmers	Kerala
8	Mercy	49	Female	Christian	U.S.	Mother (81), father passed away; husband and two children in the U.S.; sister and one brother in Kerala, second brother elsewhere in India, third brother in U.K.	Father shopkeeperz	Kerala

(*continued*)

Overview of Study Participants (*continued*)

	Name	Age*	Gender	Religion	Country of residence	Family	Parents' occupation (source of income)	Field sites/ events
9	Viju	29	Male	Church-going Hindu	U.K.	Mother (52) and father (60), brother and his family, parents-in-law in Kerala	Parents shopkeepers	Kerala
10	Thomas	28	Female	Hindu	Canada (planned)	Mother (56), father (67); sister nurse in Canada, previously Singapore	Unknown	Kerala
11	Nisha	27	Female	Christian— Orthodox Syrian	Kuwait	Father, mother (in their 50s), brother in Kerala	Unknown	Kerala
12	Anju	24	Female	Christian— Orthodox Syrian	Kuwait (planned)	Mother (50), father (52), older sister in Saudi Arabia, younger brother student in another Indian state	Father a photographer, mother a chemist, landowners	Kerala
13	Matthew	28	Male	Christian— Orthodox Syrian	Australia	Mother, father (in their 50s), younger sister	Small-scale farmers	Kerala
Parents/parents-in-law only								
14	Alice	71	Female	Christian— Orthodox Syrian	Australia	Widow, daughter nurse in Australia, son working in UAE	Unknown	Kerala

Overview of Study Participants (*continued*)

	Name	Age*	Gender	Religion	Country of residence	Family	Parents' occupation (source of income)	Field sites/ events
15	Manju	70	Female	Christian— Orthodox Syrian	Bahrain	Widow, daughter nurse in Bahrain	Unknown	Kerala
16	Sosha	53	Female	Christian Syrian Orthodox	U.K., UAE, South Africa	Husband (61), three daughters nurses abroad with own families	Father an electrician	Kerala
17	Silvia	48	Female	Christian— Pentecostal	UAE	Living alone, daughter-in-law and son in UAE, daughter nurse in Andaman Islands	Unknown	Kerala
Children only								
18	Anthony	28	Male	Christian— Orthodox Syrian	U.K., Australia	Father deceased in 2015, mother (61) and grandmother (95) living together in Kerala; brother in another Indian state	Mother a retired veterinarian, father an office worker	Kerala
19	Romy	26	Female	Christian— Orthodox Syrian	Australia	Mother (63), father (66), brother working in Dubai	Father used to work in Dubai	Texting
20	Ela	45	Female	Christian	UAE	Husband, two children; parents deceased	Unknown	Kerala

(continued)

Overview of Study Participants (*continued*)

	Name	Age*	Gender	Religion	Country of residence	Family	Parents' occupation (source of income)	Field sites/events
22	Monu	26	Male	Christian—Orthodox Syrian	New Zealand (planned)	Mother and father (in early 50s), younger sister in Kerala	Father working (occupation unknown)	Kerala
23	Ashu	50	Female	Christian—Orthodox Syrian	Oman, previously Malaysia	Sister nurse and two brothers in UAE; husband, three children, and mother (80s) living with deceased brother's wife in Kerala, father deceased; mother-in-law (80s)	Father on temporary jobs, small-scale farming	Oman
24	Sunni	57	Female	Christian—Orthodox Syrian	UAE	Son, daughter (nurse), husband in Kerala, one daughter with her in UAE; mother living with brother's family, father and parents-in-law deceased	Small-scale farming	UAE
25	Benny	31	Male	Christian—Orthodox Syrian	Oman	Wife a nurse in Oman; mother and younger brother in Kerala, father deceased	Unknown	Oman

Overview of Study Participants (continued)

	Name	Age*	Gender	Religion	Country of residence	Family	Parents' occupation (source of income)	Field sites/ events
26	Meena	53	Female	Christian—Orthodox Syrian	Oman	Parents deceased; two children with husband and mother-in-law in Kerala; brother in UAE	Unknown	Oman
27	Sona	30	Female	Christian—Orthodox Syrian	Oman	Mother, father, younger sister in Kerala; husband and two small children in Oman	Unknown	Oman
28	Neethu	30	Female	Christian—Orthodox Syrian	Oman	Husband and two young children in Oman; elder sister in U.S., father (52) and mother (52) living with younger brother, father-in-law (61) and mother-in-law (58) in Kerala	Unknown	Oman
29	Margie	27	Female	Christian—Orthodox Syrian	Australia	Mother, father (in their 50s), two younger sisters in Kerala	Unknown	Kerala
30	Abraham	26	Male	Christian—Orthodox Syrian	U.K.	Mother, father, younger sister in Kerala	Unknown	Kerala

(continued)

Overview of Study Participants (*continued*)

	Name	Age*	Gender	Religion	Country of residence	Family	Parents' occupation (source of income)	Field sites/ events
31	Pia	28	Female	Christian—Orthodox Syrian	Germany	Mother, father in Kerala; husband working in Dubai, young daughter with maternal grandparents	Unknown	Texting via WhatsApp
32	Feni	32	Female	Christian—Orthodox Syrian	Germany	Mother, father, younger sister a nurse in Germany	Unknown	Phone, texting, and audio messages via WhatsApp
33	Aaron	31	Male	Church-going Hindu	U.K.	Only son; mother (60), father (68)	Father assistant manager in a company	Video call via WhatsApp
Retired nurses, returned migrants								
34	Patti	65	Female	Christian—Orthodox Syrian	U.S.	Living with husband; daughter in U.S.	Remittances and pension	Kerala
35	Roby	68	Female	Christian—Orthodox Syrian	U.S.	Living with husband; two sons in U.S.	Remittances and pension	Kerala

Overview of Study Participants (*continued*)

	Name	Age*	Gender	Religion	Country of residence	Family	Parents' occupation (source of income)	Field sites/ events
36	Janice	63	Female	Christian—Orthodox Syrian	U.S.	Widow; two sons in U.S.	Remittances and pension	Kerala
37	Thalia	72	Female	Christian—Mathoma	U.S., UAE	Widow; son in UAE, daughter in U.S.; two sisters nurses in U.S., one sister nurse in Kuwait, and one sister married in Kerala	Remittances and pension	Kerala
38	Aly	71	Female	Christian—Roman Catholic	Germany	Living with husband; son in Abu Dhabi, daughter-in-law nurse; daughter in Kerala	Remittances and pension	Kerala

*AGE at the time of the interview.

**I note where I met the children as well as their parents, or only children or parents.

NOTES

CHAPTER 1 ENACTING CARE

1. All personal names and some names of places are pseudonyms.
2. At the time of my research, the number of people over 60 years of age was 962 million globally, and this is expected to double by 2050; the process of population aging is the most advanced in Europe and North America, where older adults account for 35 percent and 28 percent of the population, respectively (United Nations 2017b).
3. In 2013, there were 232 million international migrants, a rise of 50 percent from 1990 (United Nations 2013). In 2017, 17 million people who were born in India lived abroad (United Nations 2017a). India is the very top country in the world in terms of remittances, with migrants sending USD 69 billion to their relatives in India in 2015 (Connor 2017).
4. For examples, see Pols (2012), Nielsen (2015), and Obasola and colleagues (2015).
5. See more on enacting and perspectivism in Mol (1999), Latour (2005), Pols (2005), Law and Lien (2018), and de Castro (2019), and compare Kleinman (1988).
6. Perhaps as a consequence of coming into contact with STS (Miller 2005; Callon 2005), the acknowledgment that technologies and people shape each other is also noticeable in the more recent development of material culture studies (e.g., Miller et al. 2016).
7. STS scholars examining the problem of anthropocene have also noted that heterogenous relationships are not exactly symmetrical, and the impacts of humans on other, human or nonhuman entities are not to be underestimated or even concealed by emphasizing the constant emergence of ontologies through practices (Bonelli and Walford 2021).

CHAPTER 2 CRAFTING THE FIELD

1. According to the 2011 Census, the population of Kerala is 33.4 million people, expected to increase to 35.8 million people by 2021 (Government of India 2011). Geographically, Kerala covers almost 39,000 square kilometers; it is divided into fourteen districts, with its capital city being Thiruvananthapuram, also called Trivandrum (Government of Kerala 2021).
2. According to the Government of India Census (2011), almost 55 percent of Kerala's population are Hindu, over 26 percent Muslim (concentrated in northern Kerala), over 18 percent Christian (concentrated in southern Kerala), and less than 1 percent are Sikh, Buddhist, Jain, or other religions. Most of the Christians are Syrian (70 percent), followed by Roman Catholics (13 percent), members of the Church of South India (CSI) and Pentecostal Churches (around 4 percent each), and other denominations.
3. In Hinduism, Brahmins are considered priests and teachers; the other major castes, from highest to lowest, are the Kshatriya (warriors and princes), Vaisya (farmers or merchants), and Shudra (servants and sharecroppers). However, in Kerala this system is less rigid because Kshatriyas and Vaisyas were historically rare; the caste hierarchy became further complicated by the introduction of Syrian Christianity (Thomas 2018; see also Osella and Osella 2006).
4. See, for example, Abraham (2002), Dalrymple (2002), Sprague (2002), and various news pieces (e.g., *The Week* Staff 2020). For a critical examination of Kerala's religious exceptionalism, see Thomas (2018), and for religious conflicts in India, including anti-Christian opposition, see Bauman (2013).

5. Roman and Syrian Christians in Kerala differ in their use of language (the Roman liturgical language is Latin, and Syrian Christians use Malayalam) and the origin of their central leader. Roman Catholics have their head (the Pope) in Rome, Italy, whereas the headquarters of the Syrian Christian head (the Patriarch) is in Damascus, Syria, but was transferred to Lebanon for safety reasons after terrorist attacks in 2018. For an organizational structure of the Syrian Christian Orthodox Church from Kerala, see George (2005, 220–223).

6. The term "Dalits" (also known as untouchables or Harijan) refers to members of a wide range of low-caste Hindu groups and any person outside the caste system. Deemed offensive, the term was officially declared illegal in 1949 and was replaced with Scheduled Caste. *Encyclopaedia Britannica Online*, s.v. "Untouchable," last updated October 27, 2022, https://www.britannica.com/topic/untouchable.

7. In 2011, more than 27,000 nurses were registered in Kerala, and as many as 80 percent of nurses in cities like Delhi came from Kerala (Kodoth and Jacob 2013). Precise numbers of graduating nurses in India are difficult to establish due to the questionable reliability of data about the education of health-care workers (Walton-Roberts et al. 2017, 18). See also George (2005), Nair (2012), Percot (2006, 2016), and Percot and Rajan (2007).

8. This is significantly better from the national literacy average of 78 percent, with a 15 percent difference between men and women (Manoj 2020).

9. For a detailed examination of women's position among Syrian Christians in Kerala and abroad, see George (2005), Thomas (2018), and Abraham (2004).

10. For an ethnographic study of suicide among highly educated young people in Kerala, see Chua (2014).

11. For a detailed account of Namboodiri Brahmins, their history, and their current status in Kerala, see Gallo (2017).

12. For ethnographic studies of the Indian diaspora, see Rutten and Patel (2003) for the United Kingdom; Lamb (2009) and Das (2012) for the United States; and Vora (2013) for the United Arab Emirates (UAE).

13. The Philippines is a famous example of a country that produces nurses as a human capital for export (Yeates 2009). The case of Filipino migrants has been extensively described ethnographically and theorized within the literature on global care chains (Amrith 2017; Cabalquinto 2022; Choy 2003; McKay 2016; Parreñas 2001, 2008).

14. See Gallo (2018), Das Gupta (2009), Prescott and Nichter (2014), Nair and Healey (2006), and George (2015). Internal and international migration is common among Indians of all socioeconomic and religious backgrounds. For ethnographies on Indian migrants from other contexts, see Lamb (2009), Bomhoff (2011), Bailey, Hallard, and James (2018), and Voigt-Graf (2005).

15. See https://www.helpageindia.org/wp-content/uploads/2020/02/digital-literacy-pdf.pdf, accessed December 22, 2022.

16. See the appendix for more information about the people included in this study.

CHAPTER 3   STRUGGLING WITH ABANDONMENT

1. *Oxford English Dictionary Online*, s.v. "Abandon, v." Oxford: Oxford University Press. https://www.oed.com/view/Entry/70?rskey=UTHSFO&result=3#eid. In Malayalam, "to abandon" translates as ഉപേക്ഷിക്കാൻ (*upēkṣikkān*), with several close synonyms. For an etymological investigation of the term *abandonment* in English, see Salerno (2003, 3–4).

2. In 2017, India had around 125 million people above 60 years of age, or 9.4 percent of the population; this number is expected to increase to 316 million by 2050, or about 19 percent of the national population (United Nations 2017a). Although the World Health Organization

(2012) defines "elder people" as those who are older than 60, ethnographic literature shows that this notion is not clearly delineated or uniform across the world (e.g., Vera-Sanso 2006). Defining people as old after they reach a certain age is a relatively recent phenomenon in India. There, gerontology as a medical and social practice developed only in the 1980s. As Lawrence Cohen writes (1998, 88), before that "people did not know what a senior citizen is. . . . At that time there was no aging in India."

3. In Kerala, according to news reports from 2020, around 5 million older adults receive a pension of INR 1,300 (USD 17) per month, or INR 1,500 (USD 20) for those older than 75 (Sebastian 2020). The Government of India increased monthly pensions from INR 75 to INR 200 (USD 1 to 3) between 1995 and 2020 (Cherian 2020, vi). Around 67 percent of men and 87 percent of women do not receive any social benefits (James et al. 2013, 10). For more about pension initiatives targeting women, see van Dullemen and de Bruijn (2015).

4. In India, health expenses are mostly paid out of pocket, and the national public health expenditure remains at around 1.4 percent, well below the world average (Rao 2018).

5. According to the 2011 census, over 41 percent of the older people in India are engaging in economic activities, with this percentage being significantly higher in rural areas (Government of India 2011).

6. See Lamb (2000, 83–88) for an extensive discussion on the inappropriateness of living with a married daughter; I address this issue further in chapter 6.

7. Other sources report that old age homes appeared much earlier, in the eighteenth century, with the first records from 1782 (Rajan 2002).

8. This is despite the fact that in Western countries, too, institutionalized care is often the last resort for families, and governments increasingly encourage aging at home (e.g., Government of the Netherlands 2018). For more on the "harming" impact of Western culture on conventional Indian norms of eldercare, see Lamb (2009, 112–113; see also Lamb et al. 2017).

9. In recent decades, the practices of sevā have become transformed through diasporic life; Sarah Lamb (2009) suggests that it could now be said to include paying for an old age home or in-home care; see Lamb (2009, 193–198) for a discussion of paid care services as sevā.

10. In 2014, the Government of Kerala officially recognized 532 old age homes in the nongovernmental sector and an additional fifteen homes in the government sector (Nayar 2016, 8).

11. The Mundakapadam Mandirams Society is grounded in the Mahtoma Church, one of the many factions of the Syrian Church in Kerala. The word mandiram originates from Hindi and translates as "temple."

12. See Mundakapadam Mandirams Society, "Eventide Homes for Senior Citizens | Founded in 1977," November 2018, https://mandiram.org/senior-citizen-homes/. The prices were communicated to me via email in 2020. Lakh is a unit in the Indian numbering system that refers to 100,000.

13. See Mundakapadam Mandirams Society, "Agathi Mandiram: A Home for the Destitute | Started in 1933," November 2018, https://mandiram.org/agathi-mandiram/.

14. In her account of fictive kinship within an Indian transnational family, Brijnath (2009) argues that carers, who commonly have lower-class background, are not necessarily exploited and powerless. As their relationship develops through long-term care engagements, the family may feel obliged to support the carers, financially and otherwise, as though they were kin.

15. The website of the Mandirams Society also advertises its own Mandiram Hospital and a Palliative Home Care project, which started in 2015 after my visit.

16. See Ayyar and Khandare (2013) for more on skin color and caste discrimination in India.

17. According to 2014 exchange rates.

18. See also Vatuk's (1990) work, describing how some older adults in India decide to move to an old age home to not burden their children through co-residence.

19. See, for example, St. Mathews Home for Senior Citizens ("Paid Old Age Homes" 2021).

20. See also López and Domènech (2008) on how material agents can contribute to enacting people's autonomy in different ways.

21. For exceptions, see Jamuna (2003), Shankardass and Rajan (2018), Selim and colleagues (2018), Rajan (2022), and Rajan and Arya (2018).

CHAPTER 4   CALLING FREQUENTLY

1. Fictitious name of place.

2. By contrast, research in the early 2000s has shown that email was a popular way of communication for older parents in Italy and their adult children in Australia (Baldassar 2008). For a discussion of changing technologies over time, see Baldassar (2017).

3. See Gallo (2015) on how Malayalis use humor and irony when expressing painful emotions.

CHAPTER 5   SHIFTING DUTIES

1. The conversion rates in this section are from 2021.

2. The in-laws' demands for additional dowry cash after marriage have even been linked to "dowry-related deaths," an expression referring to deaths of young women, allegedly by suicide, following harassment over dowry; in June 2021, three such cases were reported in the news within two days (Varma 2021).

3. Similarly, other scholars have noted that in Kerala "the importance of marriage for women cannot be exaggerated" (Philips 2004, 261). According to Amali Philips (2004), the status of a single woman is intolerable, and an unmarried woman is considered *pothuppen* (a common or shared woman)—public property that men can take advantage of at any time. Women's safety is therefore intricately linked to their married status. Unsurprisingly, then, divorce is highly uncommon. According to the 2011 government census, the divorce rate for India was 0.24 percent among all married couples, with the rate in Kerala being slightly higher at 0.32 percent (Jacob and Chattopadhyay 2015).

4. See "The AksharaSilpam Project," Aksharasilpam, May 2021, https://www.kottayampublic library.org/aksharasilpam/.

5. For a further analysis of the mother-daughter relationship in South India, see Trawick (1990, 163–170).

6. In proposing the idea of kitchen as a site of care, Emily Yates-Doerr and Megan Carney (2016) note that in Latin American households, the individual was subordinate to the communal in terms of diet, and therefore individualized diets prescribed by health-care professionals were not feasible. In Kerala, however, the communal was above the individual only during liturgic occasions, which demanded specific kinds of foods. For example, at the events commemorating the death anniversaries of Mary, St. Thomas, and other important saints *pal appam* (pancakes) were served; at the yearly commemorative services of deceased parents, different cakes made of jaggery and coconut were offered (Visvanathan 1999, 170–172). Sharing food on such occasions is "an important index of solidarity of the community" among Syrian Christians (Visvanathan 1999, 171).

7. This reality fuel the discourses of international migration as tied to lower economic classes, which I discuss in chapter 3.

8. The conversion rates are from 2014, according to the reference (Johnson, Green, and Maben 2014). The amounts noted by my informants at the end of this paragraph are based on the 2018 conversion rates.

9. See Nichter (1981) for the related concept of idioms of distress.

10. Another option was TOEFL (Test of English as a Foreign Language), which was accepted for visa applications in the United States and Australia but was refused by the United Kingdom at the time of my fieldwork (Educational Testing Service, http://www.ets.org/toefl/ibt /about/, April 30, 2014). TOEFL was particularly popular for students who wished to study in the United States; only one among my interlocutors was unsure of which test to take, but all the others were studying for IELTS.

11. See, for example, Manjoorans Education Academy, "Nurses Recruitment—NHS," April 4, 2021, https://www.manjooransacademy.com/uknhs/.

12. The so-called IELTS marriages have become particularly prominent in the Indian state of Punjab in recent years (Chabba 2020).

CHAPTER 6   DOING HEALTH

1. Among the families I met, none of the parents followed their children abroad, although some children tried to convince them to do so. However, some older adults from India do follow their children abroad, and their options for doing so are shaped by different national immigration laws. See Sarah Lamb (2009) on aging parents moving from India to the United States to settle there with their children.

2. Vonage is an American VoIP provider (https://www.vonage.com/).

3. DHL is a German logistics company providing courier services.

4. As an example, in a public speech at a book fair I attended in 2014, one speaker noted how priests in India often warn of "the devil coming through the phone." The devil in this case was a metaphor for illicit romantic relationships, which could represent a danger to the institution of arranged marriage.

5. See Ahlin, Nichter, and Pillai (2016) for more on (underuse of) health insurance in India. See Ecks (2021) on how the hundreds of government-funded health insurance schemes, which have been introduced since the 2000s, are not benefitting the poor in India but instead are deepening the lack of market transparency in health care.

6. See also chapter 5 on this point.

7. To put this expense into context, in 2018–2019 the average salary for government employees in Kerala was about INR 50,000 (USD 680) per month, up from about INR 25,000 (USD 350) per month in 2011–2012 (Saikiran 2020).

CONCLUSION

1. See https://responsibletoday.in/, accessed January 8, 2023.

REFERENCES

Aboderin, Isabella. 2004. "Modernisation and Ageing Theory Revisited: Current Explanations of Recent Developing World and Historical Western Shifts in Material Family Support for Older People." *Ageing and Society* 24 (1): 29–50. https://doi.org/10.1017/S0144686X03001521.

Abraham, Abu. 2002. "Where 'Everything Is Different.'" In *Where the Rain Is Born: Writings about Kerala*, edited by Anita Nair, 96–103. New Delhi: Penguin.

Abraham, Binumol. 2004. "Women Nurses and the Notion of Their 'Empowerment.'" Thiruvananthapuram: Kerala Research Programme on Local Level Development, Centre for Development Studies.

Abrahamsson, Sebastian, Filippo Bertoni, Annemarie Mol, and Rebeca Ibáñez Martín. 2015. "Living with Omega-3: New Materialism and Enduring Concerns." *Environment and Planning D: Society and Space* 33 (1): 4–19. https://doi.org/10.1068/d14086p.

Agarwal, Bina. 1997. "'Bargaining' and Gender Relations: within and beyond the Household." *Feminist Economics* 3 (1): 51. https://doi.org/10.1080/135457097338799.

Ahlin, Tanja. 2012. "Of Food and Friendship: A Method for Understanding Eating Disorders in India." *Medische Antropologie* 24 (1): 41–56.

———. 2018. "What Keeps Maya from Eating? A Case Study of Disordered Eating from North India." *Transcultural Psychiatry* 55 (4): 551–571. https://doi.org/10.1177/13634615 18762275.

Ahlin, Tanja, and Fangfang Li. 2019. "From Field Sites to Field Events." *Medicine Anthropology Theory* 6 (2): 4931. https://doi.org/10.17157/mat.6.2.655.

Ahlin, Tanja, Mark Nichter, and Gopukrishnan Pillai. 2016. "Health Insurance in India: What Do We Know and Why Is Ethnographic Research Needed?" *Anthropology and Medicine* 23 (1): 102–124. https://doi.org/10.1080/13648470.2015.1135787.

Alshareef, Abdullah Ghaleb, Darren Wraith, Kaeleen Dingle, and Jennifer Mays. 2020. "Identifying the Factors Influencing Saudi Arabian Nurses' Turnover." *Journal of Nursing Management* 28 (5): 1030–1040. https://doi.org/10.1111/jonm.13028.

Ameerudheen, T. A. 2018. "Is the Caste System Deep-Rooted among Christians in India? A Kerala Bishop Stirs up a Hornet's Nest." *Scroll.In*, April 20, 2018. https://scroll.in/article/876000/is-the-caste-system-deep-rooted-among-christians-in-india-a-kerala-bishop-stirs-up-a-hornets-nest.

Amrith, Megha. 2017. *Caring for Strangers: Filipino Medical Workers in Asia.* Copenhagen: NIAS Press.

Anukriti, S., Nishith Prakash, and Sungoh Kwon. 2021. "The Evolution of Dowry in Rural India: 1960–2008." *World Bank Blogs*, June 30, 2021. https://blogs.worldbank.org/developmenttalk/evolution-dowry-rural-india-1960-2008.

Appadurai, Arjun. 1981. "Gastro-Politics in Hindu South Asia." *American Ethnologist* 8 (3): 494–511.

Augustine, Amala, Sanju George, and C. T. Sudhir Kumar. 2020. "Life in Old Age Homes: Reflections from God's Own Country, Kerala, India." *Journal of Geriatric Care and Research* 7 (2): 64–67.

Ayyar, Varsha, and Lalit Khandare. 2013. "Mapping Color and Caste Discrimination in Indian Society." In *The Melanin Millennium: Skin Color as 21st Century International Discourse,*

edited by Ronald E. Hall, 71–95. Dordrecht: Springer Netherlands. https://doi.org/10
.1007/978-94-007-4608-4_5.

Aziz, Riyadh Abdul. 2012. "Skype Is Still Blocked." In *Muscat Daily*, March 25, 2012. https://
web.archive.org/web/20180414065258/http://www.muscatdaily.com/Archive/Stories
-Files/Skype-is-still-blocked.

Babu, P. V., V. P. Saraphudheen, Prabha George, Praveen Kumar, and V. S. Vidya. 2019. "Gender Statistics 201–2018." Thiruvananthapuram: Department of Economics and Statistics,
Government of Kerala.

Bailey, Ajay, Jyoti Hallad, and K. S. James. 2018. "'They Had to Go': Indian Older Adults'
Experiences of Rationalizing and Compensating the Absence of Migrant Children." *Sus-
tainability* 10 (6): 1–15. https://doi.org/10.3390/su10061946.

Baldassar, Loretta. 2008. "Missing Kin and Longing to Be Together: Emotions and the Construction of Co-Presence in Transnational Relationships." *Journal of Intercultural Studies*
29 (3): 247–266. https://doi.org/10.1080/07256860802169196.

———. 2016. "De-demonizing Distance in Mobile Family Lives: Co-presence, Care Circulation and Polymedia as Vibrant Matter." *Global Networks* 16 (2): 145–163. https://doi.org
/10.1111/glob.12109.

———. 2017. "Transformations in Transnational Ageing: A Century of Caring among Italians
in Australia." In *Transnational Aging and Kin-Work*, edited by Parin Dossa and Cati Coe,
120–140. London: Rutgers University Press.

Baldassar, Loretta, and Laura Merla. 2014. *Transnational Families, Migration and the Circulation of Care: Understanding Mobility and Absence in Family Life.* London: Routledge.

Baldassar, Loretta, Mihaela Nedelcu, and Raelene Wilding. 2016. "ICT-Based Co-Presence in
Transnational Families and Communities: Challenging the Premise of Face-to-Face Proximity in Sustaining Relationships." *Global Networks* 16 (2): 133–144. https://doi.org/10.1111
/glob.12108.

Baldassar, Loretta, and Raelene Wilding. 2020. "Migration, Aging, and Digital Kinning: The
Role of Distant Care Support Networks in Experiences of Aging Well." *The Gerontologist*
60 (2): 313–321.

Barrett, Ron. 2008. *Aghor Medicine: Pollution, Death, and Healing in Northern India.* Berkeley:
University of California Press.

Barthes, Roland. 1975. "Toward a Psychosociology of Contemporary Food Consumption." In
European Diet from Preindustrial to Modern Times, edited by Elborg Foster and Robert Foster, 47–59. New York: Harper & Row.

Bauman, Chad M. 2013. "Hindu-Christian Conflict in India: Globalization, Conversion, and
the Coterminal Castes and Tribes." *Journal of Asian Studies* 72 (3): 633–653. https://doi
.org/10.1017/S0021911813000569.

Bennett, Jane. 2004. *Vibrant Matter: A Political Ecology of Things.* London: Duke University Press.

Bhalla, Vibha. 2008. "'Couch Potatoes and Super-Women': Gender, Migration, and the Emerging Discourse on Housework among Asian Indian Immigrants." *Journal of American Ethnic
History* 27 (4): 71–99.

Biju, B. L. 2013. "India: Angels Are Turning Red—Nurses' Strikes in Kerala." *Economic and
Political Weekly* 48 (51): 25–28.

Blaser, Mario, and Marisol de la Cadena. 2018. "Introduction: Pluriverse. Proposal for a World
of Many Worlds." In *A World of Many Worlds*, edited by Marisol de la Cadena and Mario
Blaser, 1–22. Durham, NC: Duke University Press.

Bomhoff, Manja. 2011. "Long-Lived Sociality: A Cultural Analysis of Middle-Class Older Persons' Social Lives in Kerala, India." PhD diss., Leiden University. http://hdl.handle.net
/1887/18139.

Bonelli, Cristóbal, and Antonia Walford. 2021. *Environmental Alterities*. Manchester: Mattering Press.

Bowker, Geoffrey C., and Susan Leigh Star. 2000. *Sorting Things Out: Classification and Its Consequences*. London: MIT Press.

Brijnath, Bianca. 2009. "Familial Bonds and Boarding Passes: Understanding Caregiving in a Transnational Context." *Identities: Global Studies in Culture and Power* 16 (1): 83–101.

———. 2014. *Unforgotten: Love and the Culture of Dementia Care in India*. London: Berghahn.

Bryceson, Deborah, and Ulla Vuorela. 2002. *The Transnational Family: New European Frontiers and Global Networks*. New York: Berg.

Cabalquinto, Earvin. 2022. *(Im)Mobile Homes: Family Life at a Distance in the Age of Mobile Media*. New York: Oxford University Press.

Cabalquinto, Earvin, and Tanja Ahlin. 2021. "Care within or out of Reach: Fantasies of Care and Connectivity in the Time of the COVID-19 Pandemic." In *Viral Loads: Anthropologies of Urgency in the Time of COVID-19*, edited by Lenore Manderson, Nancy Burke, and Ayo Wahlberg, 344–361. London: UCL Press.

Cadena, Marisol de la, Marianne E. Lien, Mario Blaser, Casper Bruun Jensen, Tess Lea, Atsuro Morita, Heather Swanson, Gro B. Ween, Paige West, and Margaret Wiener. 2015. "Anthropology and STS: Generative Interfaces, Multiple Locations." *HAU: Journal of Ethnographic Theory* 5 (1): 437–475. https://doi.org/10.14318/hau5.1.020.

Callon, Michel. 2005. "Why Virtualism Paves the Way to Political Impotence: A Reply to Daniel Miller's Critique of 'The Laws of the Market.'" *Economic Sociology: European Electronic Newsletter* 6 (2): 3–20.

Callon, Michel, and John Law. 1997. "After the Individual in Society: Lessons on Collectivity from Science, Technology and Society." *Canadian Journal of Sociology/Cahiers Canadiens de Sociologie* 22 (2): 165–182. https://doi.org/10.2307/3341747.

Carsten, Janet. 1995. "The Substance of Kinship and the Heat of the Hearth: Feeding, Personhood, and Relatedness among Malays in Pulau Langkawi." *American Ethnologist* 22 (2): 223–241. https://doi.org/10.1525/ae.1995.22.2.02a00010.

———. 2012. "Fieldwork since the 1980s: Total Immersion and Its Discontents." In *The SAGE Handbook of Social Anthropology*, edited by Richard Fardon, Oliva Harris, Trevor H. J. Marchand, Cris Shore, Veronica Strang, Richard Wilson, and Mark Nuttall, 507–518. London: SAGE London.

Chabba, Seerat. 2020. "'IELTS Marriages'—India's 'Ideal Bride' Is Proficient in English." *Deutsche Welle (DW)*, May 5, 2020. https://www.dw.com/en/ielts-marriages-indias-ideal-bride-is-proficient-in-english/a-53341947.

Chacko, Elizabeth. 2003. "Marriage, Development, and the Status of Women in Kerala, India." *Gender and Development* 11 (2): 52–59. https://doi.org/10.1080/741954317.

Chadha, Kashish. 2020. "Indian Cricketers Back 'India's Close-Knit Family Culture' to Help Mentally Cope Up with COVID-19 Crisis." *Circle of Cricket*, March 29, 2020. https://circleofcricket.com/category/Latest_news/50506/indian-cricketers-back-indias-close-knit-family-culture-to-help-mentally-cope-up-with-covid-19-crisis.

Chandran, Vivek R. 2018. "Govt to Act against Those Who Abandon Parents." *Mathrubhumi*, December 28, 2018. https://english.mathrubhumi.com/news/kerala/govt-to-act-against-those-who-abandon-parents-1.3431735.

Cherian, Mathew. 2020. *Ageing and Poverty in India*. New Delhi: Paranjoy Guha Thakurta.

Choy, Catherine Ceniza. 2003. *Empire of Care: Nursing and Migration in Filipino American History*. Durham, NC: Duke University Press.

Chua, Jocelyn Lim. 2014. *In Pursuit of the Good Life: Aspiration and Suicide in Globalizing South India*. Berkeley: University of California Press.

Cohen, Lawrence. 1998. *No Aging in India: Alzheimer's, the Bad Family, and Other Modern Things*. Berkeley: University of California Press.

Connor, Phillip. 2017. "India Is a Top Source and Destination for World's Migrants." *Pew Research Center*, March 3, 2017. https://www.pewresearch.org/fact-tank/2017/03/03/india -is-a-top-source-and-destination-for-worlds-migrants/.

Costa, Elisabetta. 2018. "Affordances-in-Practice: An Ethnographic Critique of Social Media Logic and Context Collapse." *New Media and Society* 20 (10): 3641–3656. https://doi.org /10.1177/1461444818756290.

Couldry, Nick, and Ulises A. Mejias. 2019. *The Costs of Connection: How Data Is Colonizing Human Life and Appropriating It for Capitalism. The Costs of Connection*. Stanford, CA: Stanford University Press. https://doi.org/10.1515/9781503609754.

Cowling, Jon. 2016. "A Brief History of Skype—the Peer to Peer Messaging Service." *DSP-Explorer*, February 8, 2016. https://content.dsp.co.uk/history-of-skype.

Dalal, Roshen. 2010. *Hinduism: An Alphabetical Guide*. New Delhi: Penguin.

Dalrymple, William. 2002. "In Search of Doubting Thomas." In *Where the Rain Is Born: Writings About Kerala*, edited by Anita Nair, 65–73. New Delhi: Penguin.

Das, Ashidhara. 2012. *Desi Dreams: Indian Immigrant Women Build Lives across Two Worlds*. New Delhi: Primius.

Das Gupta, Monica, Jiang Zhenghua, Li Bohua, Xie Zhenming, Woojin Chung, and Bae Hwa-Ok. 2003. "Why Is Son Preference so Persistent in East and South Asia? A Cross-Country Study of China, India and the Republic of Korea." *Journal of Development Studies* 40 (2): 153–187. https://doi.org/10.1080/00220380412331293807.

Das Gupta, Tanja. 2009. *"Real" Nurses and "Others": Racism in Nursing*. Halifax: Fernwood.

Datta, Romita. 2018. "Eldercare: Demographic Downside." *India Today*, April 26, 2018. https:// www.indiatoday.in/magazine/nation/story/20180507-branded-corporate-elderly-care -old-age-homes-1221657-2018-04-26.

De Castro, Eduardo Viveiros. 2019. "Exchanging Perspectives: The Transformation of Objects into Subjects in Amerindian Ontologies." *Common Knowledge* 25 (1–3): 21–42. https://doi .org/10.1215/0961754X-7299066.

De Jong, Willemijn. 2011. "Securing Intergenerational Kin Relationships and a House of One's Own." *Anthropology in Action* 18 (3): 10–20. https://doi.org/10.3167/aia.2011.180302.

———. 2014. "Aging and Social (In)Security in Kerala: Rethinking Research Topics and Tools." Paper presented at the Global Aging Colloquium Series, Spring 2014, Institute for European Global Studies, University of Basel, Basel, April 16. https://doi.org/10.5167/uzh -108873.

Devika, J. 2010. "Egalitarian Developmentalism, Communist Mobilization, and the Question of Caste in Kerala State, India." *Journal of Asian Studies* 69 (3): 799–820.

Devika, J., and Binitha V. Thampi. 2007. "Between 'Empowerment' and 'Liberation': The Kudumbashree Initiative in Kerala." *Indian Journal of Gender Studies* 14 (1): 33–60. https:// doi.org/10.1177/097152150601400103.

Diamond-Smith, Nadia, Nancy Luke, and Stephen McGarvey. 2008. "'Too Many Girls, Too Much Dowry': Son Preference and Daughter Aversion in Rural Tamil Nadu, India." *Culture, Health and Sexuality* 10 (7): 697–708. https://doi.org/10.1080/13691050802061665.

Doffman, Zak. 2021. "Why You Should Quit WhatsApp as Critical New Update Confirmed." *Forbes*, March 6, 2021. https://www.forbes.com/sites/zakdoffman/2021/03/06/stop-using -whatsapp-after-facebook-apple-imessage-signal-and-telegram-privacy-backlash/.

Driessen, Annelieke. 2018. "Thinking Pain." *Somatosphere*, October 1, 2018. http://somato sphere.net/2018/thinking-pain.html/.

Dutta, Upanga. 2015. "Women and Senior Citizens: The Unconnected Digital India." *DNA India*, December 26, 2015. https://www.dnaindia.com/business/report-women-and-senior-citizens-the-unconnected-digital-india-2159640.

Ecks, Stefan. 2021. "'Demand Side' Health Insurance in India: The Price of Obfuscation." *Medical Anthropology* 40 (5): 404–416. https://doi.org/10.1080/01459740.2021.1929208.

Economist Staff. 2020. "The World Desperately Needs More Nurses." *The Economist*, December 11, 2020. https://www.economist.com/graphic-detail/2020/12/11/the-world-desperately-needs-more-nurses.

Edwards, Paul. 2003. "Infrastructure and Modernity: Force, Time and Social Organization in the History of Sociotechnical Systems." In *Modernity and Technology*, edited by Thomas J. Misa, Philip Brey, and Andrew Feenberg, 185–226. London: MIT Press.

Express News Service. 2018. "Kerala Nurses' Salary Hike: High Court Restrains Government from Issuing Final Notification." *New Indian Express*, March 16, 2018. http://www.newindianexpress.com/states/kerala/2018/mar/16/kerala-nurses-salary-hike-high-court-restrains-government-from-issuing-final-notification-1787816.html.

Falkingham, Jane, Min Qin, Athina Vlachantoni, and Maria Evandrou. 2017. "Children's Migration and Lifestyle-Related Chronic Disease among Older Parents 'Left Behind' in India." *SSM—Population Health* 3 (December): 352–357. https://doi.org/10.1016/j.ssmph.2017.03.008.

Fisher, Tom H. 2004. "What We Touch, Touches Us: Materials, Affects, and Affordances." *Design Issues* 20 (4): 20–31.

Fuller, C. J. 1976. "Kerala Christians and the Caste System." *Man* 11 (1): 53–70. https://doi.org/10.2307/2800388.

Gajjala, Radhika, and Tarishi Verma. 2018. "WhatsAppified Diasporas and Transnational Circuits of Affect and Relationality." In *Appified: Culture in the Age of Apps*, edited by Jeremy Wade Morris and Sarah Murray, 205–215. Ann Arbor: University of Michigan Press.

Gallo, Ester. 2005. "Unorthodox Sisters: Gender Relations and Generational Change among Malayali Migrants in Italy." *Indian Journal of Gender Studies* 12 (3): 217–251. https://doi.org/10.1177/097152150501200204.

———. 2006. "Italy Is Not a Good Place for Men: Narratives of Places, Marriage and Masculinity among Malayali Migrants." *Global Networks* 6 (4): 357–372.

———. 2015. "The Irony of Kinship Migration and the Control of Emotions among Malayalis." *Emotion, Space and Society* 16 (August): 108–115. https://doi.org/10.1016/j.emospa.2014.12.001.

———. 2017. *The Fall of Gods: Memory, Kinship, and Middle Classes in South India*. New Delhi: Oxford University Press.

———. 2018. "A Broken Chain? Colonial History, Middle-Class Indian Migrants and Intergenerational Ambivalence." *International Journal of Comparative Sociology* 60 (1–2): 37–54. https://doi.org/10.1177/0020715218815728.

———. 2021. "Kinship as a 'Public Fiction': Substance and Emptiness in South Indian Inter-Caste and Inter-Religious Families." *Contemporary South Asia* 29 (1): 81–96.

Gallo, Ester, and Francesca Scrinzi. 2016. *Migration, Masculinities and Reproductive Labour*. London: Palgrave Macmillan.

Gamburd, Michele R. 2000. *The Kitchen Spoon's Handle: Transnationalism and Sri Lanka's Migrant Housemaids*. New York: Cornell University Press.

———. 2008. "Milk Teeth and Jet Planes: Kin Relations in Families of Sri Lanka's Transnational Domestic Servants." *City and Society* 20 (1): 5–31. https://doi.org/10.1111/j.1548-744X.2008.00003.x.

Gardner, William, David States, and Nicholas Bagley. 2020. "The Coronavirus and the Risks to the Elderly in Long-Term Care." *Journal of Aging and Social Policy* 32 (4–5): 310–315. https://doi.org/10.1080/08959420.2020.1750543.

Garfinkel, Harold. (1967) 1990. *Studies in Ethnomethodology.* Cambridge: Polity Press.

Genovese, Barbara J. 2004. "Thinking inside the Box: The Art of Telephone Interviewing." *Field Methods* 16 (2): 215–226. https://doi.org/10.1177/1525822X04263329.

George, Sheba Mariam. 2005. *When Women Come First: Gender and Class in Transnational Migration.* Los Angeles: University of California Press.

———. 2015. "'Real Nursing Work' Versus 'Charting and Sweet Talking': The Challenges of Incorporation in US Urban Healthcare Settings for Indian Immigrant Nurses." In *Bodies across Borders; The Global Circulation of Body Parts, Medical Tourists and Professionals,* edited by Bronwyn Parry, Beth Greenhough, and Isabel Dyck, 133–153. London: Ashgate.

Goelitz, Ann. 2003. "When Accessibility Is an Issue: Telephone Support Groups for Caregivers." *Smith College Studies in Social Work* 73 (3): 385–394.

Goody, Jack. (1982) 1996. *Cooking, Cuisine and Class: A Study in Comparative Sociology.* Cambridge: Cambridge University Press.

Gorham, Bradley W. 1999. "Stereotypes in the Media: So What?" *Howard Journal of Communications* 10 (4): 229–247. https://doi.org/10.1080/106461799246735.

Government of India. 2011. "Census of India: Population by Religious Community." New Delhi: Office of the Registrar General & Census, Ministry of Home Affairs.

Government of Kerala. 2021. "About District—Kottayam District." 2021. https://kottayam.nic .in/about-district/.

Government of the Netherlands. 2018. "Living Independently for Longer—Care and Support at Home—government.nl." Living Independently for Longer. The Hague: Ministerie van Algemene Zaken. https://www.government.nl/topics/care-and-support-at-home/living -independently-for-longer.

Gregory, Chris. 2011. "Skinship: Touchability as a Virtue in East-Central India." *HAU: Journal of Ethnographic Theory* 1 (1): 179–209. https://doi.org/10.14318/hau1.1.007.

Grover, Sandeep, Swapnajeet Sahoo, Aseem Mehra, Ajit Avasthi, Adarsh Tripathi, Alka Subramanyan, Amrit Pattojoshi, et al. 2020. "Psychological Impact of COVID-19 Lockdown: An Online Survey from India." *Indian Journal of Psychiatry* 62 (4): 354–362. https://doi .org/10.4103/psychiatry.IndianJPsychiatry_427_20.

Haenssgen, Marco. 2019. "Manifestations, Drivers, and Frictions of Mobile Phone Use in Low- and Middle-Income Settings: A Mixed Methods Analysis of Rural India and China." *Journal of Development Studies* 55 (8): 1834–1858. https://doi.org/10.1080/00220388.2018 .1453605.

Hansen, Thomas Blom. 2001. "Bridging the Gulf: Global Horizons, Mobility and Local Identity among Muslims in Mumbai." In *Community, Empire and Migration: South Asians in Diaspora,* edited by Crispin Bates, 261–285. London: Palgrave Macmillan. https://doi.org /10.1057/9780333977293_11.

Haraway, Donna. 1991. "Situated Knowledges: The Science Question in Feminism and the Privilege of Partial Perspective." In *Simians, Cyborgs, and Women: The Reinvention of Women,* edited by Donna Haraway, 183–202. London: Free Association Books.

Harbers, Hans, Annemarie Mol, and Alice Stollmeyer. 2002. "Food Matters: Arguments for an Ethnography of Daily Care." *Theory, Culture and Society* 19 (5/6): 207–226.

HelpAge India. 2020. "Elderly Empowerment in the Digital Age." HelpAge India, February 2020. https://www.helpageindia.org/elderly-empowerment-in-the-digital-age-2/.

HelpAge International. 2021. "Bearing the Brunt: The Impact of COVID-19 on Older People in Low- and Middle-Income Countries—Insights from 2020." London: HelpAge International.

Hindustan Times Correspondent, Mumbai. 2011. "280 Nurses Go on Strike after Colleague's Suicide." *Hindustan Times*, October 20, 2011. https://www.hindustantimes.com/mumbai /280-nurses-go-on-strike-after-colleague-s-suicide/story-ot9X9NGkcoiUbzrFKdDCuM .html.

Hochschild, Arlie Russell. 2000. "Global Care Chains and Emotional Surplus Value." In *On the Edge: Living with Global Capitalism*, edited by T. Giddens and W. Hutton, 130–146. London: SAGE.

Hoogsteyns, Maartje. 2008. "Artefact Mens: Een Interdisciplinair Onderzoek Naar Het Debat over Materialiteit Binnen de Material Culture Studies." [Artifact Human: An Interdisciplinary Research on the Debate on Materiality within the Material Culture Studies.] Amsterdam: University of Amsterdam.

Hromadžić, Azra. 2018. "'Where Were They until Now?' Aging, Care, and Abandonment in a Bosnian Town." In *Care across Distance: Ethnographic Explorations of Aging and Migration*, edited by Azra Hromadžić and Monika Palmberger, 156–170. Oxford: Berghahn.

Hromadžić, Azra, and Monika Palmberger, eds. 2018. *Care across Distance: Ethnographic Explorations of Aging and Migration.* Oxford: Berghahn.

Human Rights Watch. 2020. "COVID-19: Unblock Voice Over IP Platforms in Gulf." *Human Rights Watch*, April 7, 2020. https://www.hrw.org/news/2020/04/07/covid-19-unblock -voice-over-ip-platforms-gulf.

International Institute for Population Sciences. 2017. "National Family Health Survey (NFHS-4), 2015–2016: India." Mumbai: International Institute for Population Sciences (IIPS) and ICF.

International Labour Organization. 2018. "India Labour Migration Update 2018." New Delhi: International Labour Organization.

ITP Staff. 2012. "Oman Government Unblocks Some VoIP Services—ITP.Net." *ITP.net*, April 10, 2012. https://www.itp.net/news/588597-oman-government-unblocks-some-voip -services.

Jacob, Suraj, and Sreeparna Chattopadhyay. 2015. "Marriage Dissolution in India." *Economic and Political Weekly* 51 (33): 7–8.

Jain, Samidha. 2021. "Indians Most Active on WhatsApp with 390.1 Million Monthly Active Users in 2020." *Forbes India*, August 27, 2021. https://www.forbesindia.com/article/news -by-numbers/indians-most-active-on-whatsapp-with-3901-million-monthly-active-users -in-2020/70059/1.

James, K. S. T. S. Syamala, Supriya Verma, Sajini B. Nair, L. Shylaja, S. Sureshkumar, and K. R. Anithakumari. 2013. "The Status of Elderly in Kerala, 2011." Institute for Social and Economic Change (ISEC) Bangalore, Tata Institute of Social Sciences (TISS), and United Nations Population Fund (UNFPA). https://india.unfpa.org/sites/default/files /pub-pdf/BKPAI_Kerala_26thDec2013Final-Lowres.pdf.

Jamuna, Duvvuru. 2003. "Issues of Elder Care and Elder Abuse in the Indian Context." *Journal of Aging and Social Policy* 15 (2–3): 125–142. https://doi.org/10.1300/J031v15n02_08.

Jeffrey, Robin. 2004. "Legacies of Matriliny: The Place of Women and the 'Kerala Model.'" *Pacific Affairs* 77 (4): 647–664.

———. 2016. *Politics, Women and Well-Being: How Kerala Became "a Model."* Basingstoke, United Kingdom: Palgrave Macmillan.

Jeffrey, Robin, and Assa Doron. 2013. *The Great Indian Phone Book: How Cheap Mobile Phones Change Business, Politics and Daily Life.* London: Hurst. https://www.hurstpublishers.com /book/the-great-indian-phonebook/.

Jensen, Casper Bruun, and Brit Ross Winthereik. 2013. *Monitoring Movements in Development Aid: Recursive Partnerships and Infrastructures.* Cambridge, MA: MIT Press.

Johnson, Sonali E., Judith Green, and Jill Maben. 2014. "A Suitable Job?: A Qualitative Study of Becoming a Nurse in the Context of a Globalizing Profession in India." *International Journal of Nursing Studies* 51 (5): 734–743. https://doi.org/10.1016/j.ijnurstu.2013.09.009.

Joju, Jacob, and P. K. Manoj. 2019. "Digital Kerala: A Study of the ICT: Initiatives in Kerala State." *International Journal of Research in Engineering, IT and Social Sciences* 9: 692–703.

Joseph, Jeethu, dir. 2015. *Life of Josutty*. India: Eros International. DVD video.

Joseph, Raju, dir. 1993. *Dollar*. Dubai: RAFA. VHS video.

Karagiannidis, C., S. Kluge, R. Riessen, M. Krakau, T. Bein, and U. Janssens. 2019. "Auswirkungen des Pflegepersonalmangels auf die intensivmedizinische Versorgungskapazität in Deutschland." [Impact of Nursing Staff Shortage on Intensive Care Medicine Capacity in Germany.] *Medizinische Klinik, Intensivmedizin Und Notfallmedizin* 114 (4): 327–333. https://doi.org/10.1007/s00063-018-0457-3.

Karner, Tracy X. 1998. "Professional Caring: Homecare Workers as Fictive Kin." *Journal of Aging Studies* 12 (1): 69–82.

Khan, Mohd Imran, and Valetheeswaran Chinnakkannu. 2020. "International Remittances and Private Healthcare in Kerala, India." *Migration Letters* 17 (3): 445–460.

Kilkey, Majella, and Laura Merla. 2014. "Situating Transnational Families' Care-giving Arrangements: The Role of Institutional Contexts." *Global Networks* 14 (2): 210–229.

Kleinman, Arthur. 1988. *The Illness Narratives: Suffering, Healing and the Human Condition*. New York: Basic Books.

Kodoth, Praveena, and Tina Kuriakose Jacob. 2013. "International Mobility of Nurses from Kerala (India) to the EU: Prospects and Challenges with Special Reference to the Netherlands and Denmark." CARIM-India RR2013/9. San Domenico di Fiesole (FI): European University Institute, Robert Schuman Centre for Advanced Studies.

Kowalski, Julia. 2016. "Ordering Dependence: Care, Disorder, and Kinship Ideology in North Indian Antiviolence Counseling." *American Ethnologist* 43 (1): 63–75. https://doi.org/10.1111/amet.12263.

Krishnamoorthy, Ennapadam S. 2015. "Home Alone! How We Use Integrative Medicine to Provide Home Based Rehabilitation." *LinkedIn*, December 27, 2015. https://www.linkedin.com/pulse/home-alone-how-we-use-integrative-medicine-provide-krishnamoorthy.

Lamb, Sarah. 1997. "The Making and Unmaking of Persons: Notes on Aging and Gender in North India." *Ethos* 25 (3): 279–302. https://www.jstor.org/stable/640667.

———. 2000. *White Saris and Sweet Mangoes: Aging, Gender, and Body in North India*. Berkeley: University of California Press.

———. 2009. *Aging and the Indian Diaspora: Cosmopolitan Families in India and Abroad*. Bloomington: Indiana University Press.

———. 2013. "Personhood, Appropriate Dependence, and the Rise of Elder-Care Institutions in India." In *Transitions and Transformations: Cultural Perspectives on Aging and the Life Course*, edited by C. Lynch and J. Danely, 171–187. Oxford: Berghahn.

Lamb, Sarah, Jessica Robbins-Ruszkowski, Anna Corwin, Toni Calasanti, and Neal King. 2017. *Successful Aging as a Contemporary Obsession: Global Perspectives*. New Brunswick, NJ: Rutgers University Press. https://muse.jhu.edu/book/52075.

Larkin, Brian. 2008. *Signal and Noise: Media, Infrastructure, and Urban Culture in Nigeria*. London: Duke University Press.

Latour, Bruno. 2005. *Reassembling the Social: An Introduction to Actor-Network-Theory*. Oxford: Oxford University Press.

Law, John. 2002. "On Hidden Heterogeneities: Complexity, Formalism, and Aircraft Design." In *Complexities: Social Studies of Knowledge Practices*, edited by J. Law and A. Mol, 116–141. Durham, North Carolina: Duke University Press.

———. 2009. "Actor Network Theory and Material Semiotics." In *The New Blackwell Companion to Social Theory*, edited by B. S. Turner, 141–158. Oxford: Blackwell.

Law, John, and Marianne E. Lien. 2018. "Denaturalizing Nature." In *A World of Many Worlds*, edited by Marisol de la Cadena and Mario Blaser, 131–172. Durham, NC: Duke University Press.

Licoppe, Christian. 2004. "'Connected' Presence: The Emergence of a New Repertoire for Managing Social Relationships in a Changing Communication Technoscape." *Environment and Planning D: Society and Space* 22 (1): 135–156. https://doi.org/10.1068/d323t.

Licoppe, Christian, and Zbigniew Smoreda. 2005. "Are Social Networks Technologically Embedded? How Networks Are Changing Today with Changes in Communication Technology." *Social Networks* 27 (4): 317–335. https://doi.org/10.1016/j.socnet.2004.11.001.

López, Daniel, and Miquel Domènech. 2008. "Embodying Autonomy in a Home Telecare Service." Supplement, *Sociological Review* 56 (2): 181–195. https://doi.org/10.1111/j.1467-954X.2009.00822.x.

Madianou, Mirca, and Daniel Miller. 2012. *Migration and New Media: Transnational Families and Polymedia*. Abingdon, United Kingdom: Routledge.

Mahapatro, Sandhya, Ajay Bailey, K. S. James, and Inge Hutter. 2015. "Remittances and Household Expenditure Patterns in India and Selected States." *Migration and Development* 6 (1): 83–101.

Manderson, Lenore. 1986. "Introduction: The Anthropology of Food in Oceania and Southeast Asia." In *Shared Wealth and Symbols: Food, Culture and Society in Oceania and Southeast Asia*, 1–25. New York: Cambridge University Press.

Manderson, Lenore, and Carolyn Smith-Morris, eds. 2010. *Chronic Conditions, Fluid States: Chronicity and the Anthropology of Illness*. London: Rutgers University Press.

Manoj, C. L. 2020. "At 96.2%, Kerala Tops Literacy Rate Chart; Andhra Pradesh Worst Performer at 66.4%." *Economic Times*, September 8, 2020. https://economictimes.indiatimes.com/news/politics-and-nation/at-96-2-kerala-tops-literacy-rate-chart-andhra-pradesh-worst-performer-at-66-4/articleshow/77978682.cms.

Marcus, George E. 1995. "Ethnography in/of the World System: The Emergence of Multi-Sited Ethnography." *Annual Review of Anthropology* 24 (1): 95–117. https://doi.org/10.1146/annurev.an.24.100195.000523.

Marriott, McKim. 1968. "Caste Ranking and Food Transactions: A Matrix Analysis." In *Structure and Change in Indian Society*, edited by M. Singer and B. S. Cohn, 133–171. New York: Wenner-Gren Foundation for Anthropological Research, Inc.

Massey, Doreen. 2003. "Imagining the Field." In *Using Social Theory: Thinking through Research*, edited by M. Pryke, G. Rose, and S. Whatmore, 71–88. London: SAGE.

Mathews, V. K. 2018. "Kerala Best Suited for Digital Era." *Deccan Chronicle*, March 21, 2018. https://www.deccanchronicle.com/nation/in-other-news/210318/kerala-best-suited-for-digital-era.html.

Mauss, Marcel. 1969. *The Gift: Forms and Functions of Exchange in Archaic Societies*. London: Routledge and Kegan Paul.

McKay, Deirdre. 2016. *An Archipelago of Care: Filipino Migrants and Global Networks*. Bloomington: Indiana University Press.

McKetta, Isla. 2019. "Analyzing India's 4G Availability: Including a Look at the 15 Largest Cities." *Speedtest Stories & Analysis*, February 11, 2019. https://www.speedtest.net/insights/blog/india-4g-availability-2019/.

Medacs Healthcare. 2019. "How NMC Rule Changes to IELTS Writing Are Good News for International Nurses." *Medacs Healthcare*, May 16, 2019. https://www.medacs.com/blog/how-nmc-rule-changes-to-ielts-writing-are-good-news-for-international-nurses.

Menon, Priya. 2018. "Senior Citizens Get a Crash Course in Using Smartphones." *Times of India*, May 24, 2018. http://timesofindia.indiatimes.com/articleshow/64296179.cms.

Metz, Cade. 2009. "Oman Cuffs 212 for Selling VoIP Calls." *The Register*, November 20, 2009. https://www.theregister.com/2009/11/20/oman_and_voip/.

Miller, Daniel. 1998. "Introduction: Why Some Things Matter." In *Material Cultures: Why Some Things Matter*, edited by D. Miller, 3–21. London: UCL Press.

Miller, Daniel. 2005. "Reply to Michel Callon." *Economic Sociology: European Electronic Newsletter* 6 (3): 3–13. https://www.econstor.eu/bitstream/10419/155849/1/vol06-no03-a2.pdf.

Miller, Daniel, Elisabetta Costa, Nell Haynes, Tom McDonald, Razvan Nicolescu, Jolynna Sinanan, Juliano Spyer, Shriram Venkatraman, and Xinyuan Wang. 2016. *How the World Changed Social Media*. London: UCL Press.

Mines, Mattison. 1994. *Public Faces, Private Lives: Community and Individuality in South India*. Berkeley: University of California Press.

Mol, Annemarie. 1999. "Ontological Politics. A Word and Some Questions." Supplement, *Sociological Review* 47 (1): 74–89. https://doi.org/10.1111/j.1467-954X.1999.tb03483.x.

———. 2002. *The Body Multiple: Ontology in Medical Practice*. Durham, NC: Duke University Press.

———. 2008. *The Logic of Care: Health and the Problem of Patient Choice*. London: Routledge.

Mol, Annemarie, and Anita Hardon. 2020. "What COVID-19 May Teach Us about Interdisciplinarity." *BMJ Global Health* 5: e004375. https://doi.org/10.1136/bmjgh-2020-004375.

Mol, Annemarie, Ingunn Moser, and Jeannette Pols, eds. 2010. *Care in Practice: On Tinkering in Clinics, Homes and Farms*. Bielefeld, Germany: Transcript Verlag.

Morgan, D. 2011. *Rethinking Family Practices*. Basingstoke, United Kingdom: Palgrave Macmillan.

Mukhopadhyay, Swapna, ed. 2007. *The Enigma of the Kerala Woman: A Failed Promise of Literacy*. New Delhi: Social Science Press.

Muruvelil, Venu. 2015. "Old Parents Dumped Like Waste: Abuse of Senior Citizens on the Rise in Kerala." *Folomojo*, November 17, 2015. http://www.folomojo.com/old-parents-dumped-like-waste-abuse-of-senior-citizens-on-the-rise-in-kerala/.

Nair, Anita, ed. 2002. *Where the Rain Is Born: Writings about Kerala*. New Delhi: Penguin.

Nair, Sreelekha. 2012. *Moving with the Times: Gender, Status and Migration of Nurses in India*. New Delhi: Routledge.

Nair, Sreelekha, and Madelaine Healey. 2006. *A Profession on the Margins: Status Issues in Indian Nursing*. New Delhi: Center for Women's Development Studies.

Nair, Sreelekha, and Marie Percot. 2007. *Transcending Boundaries: Indian Nurses in Internal and International Migration*. New Delhi: Centre for Women's Development Studies.

Nair, Vinod. 2016. "Only Oman-Based VoIP Calls Legal." *Oman Daily Observer*, April 17, 2016. https://www.pressreader.com/oman/oman-daily-observer/20160417/page/1.

Narasimhan, Haripriya, Mahati Chittem, and Pooja Purang. 2021. "Pandemic Times in a WhatsApp-Ed Nation: Gender Ideologies in India during COVID-19." In *Viral Loads: Anthropologies of Urgency in the Time of COVID-19*, edited by Lenore Manderson, Nancy Burke, and Ayo Wahlberg, 362–383. London: UCL Press.

Narayana, M. R. 2019. "Old Age Pension Scheme in India: Distributional Impacts." *South Asia Research* 39 (2): 143–165. https://doi.org/10.1177/0262728019842016.

Nayar, P.K.B. 2016. *Manual on Old Age Homes*. Thiruvananthapuram, India: Centre for Gerontological Studies Kesavadasapuram.

Nedelcu, Mihaela, and Malika Wyss. 2016. "'Doing Family' through ICT-Mediated Ordinary Co-Presence: Transnational Communication Practices of Romanian Migrants in Switzerland." *Global Networks* 16 (2): 202–218. https://doi.org/10.1111/glob.12110.

Nguyen, Hien Thi, Loretta Baldassar, Raelene Wilding, and Lukasz Krzyzowski. 2021. "Researching Older Vietnam-Born Migrants at a Distance: The Role of Digital Kinning." In *Qualitative and Digital Research in Times of Crisis: Methods, Reflexivity, and Ethics,* edited by Helen Kara and Su-ming Khoo, 184–200. Bristol, United Kingdom: Policy Press.

Nichter, Mark. 1981. "Idioms of Distress: Alternatives in the Expression of Psychosocial Distress: A Case Study from South India." *Culture, Medicine and Psychiatry* 5 (4): 379–408. https://doi.org/10.1007/BF00054782.

Nielsen, Karen Dam. 2015. "Involving Patients with E-Health—The Dialogic Dynamics of Information Filtration Work." *Science and Technology Studies* 28 (2): 29–52. https://doi.org/10.23987/sts.55349.

Obasola, Oluwaseun Ireti, Iyabo Mabawonku, and Ikeoluwa Lagunju. 2015. "A Review of E-Health Interventions for Maternal and Child Health in Sub-Sahara Africa." *Maternal and Child Health Journal* 19 (8): 1813–1824. https://doi.org/10.1007/s10995-015-1695-0.

Okely, Judith. 2007. "Fieldwork Embodied." Supplement, *Sociological Review* 55 (S1): 65–79. https://doi.org/10.1111/j.1467-954X.2007.00693.x.

Osella, Caroline, and Filippo Osella. 2006. *Men and Masculinities in South India.* London: Anthem Press.

———. 2008. "Nuancing the Migrant Experience: Perspectives from Kerala, South India." In *Transnational South Asians: The Making of a Neo-Diaspora,* edited by S. Koshy and R. Radhakrishnan, 146–178. New Delhi: Oxford University Press.

Osella, Filippo, and Caroline Osella. 2007. "'I Am Gulf': The Production of Cosmopolitanism in Kozhikode, Kerala, India." In *Struggling with History: Islam and Cosmopolitanism in the Western Indian Ocean,* edited by Edward Simpson and Kai Kress, 323–356. New York: Columbia University Press, 2007.

Pahwa, Aashish. 2021. "The History Of WhatsApp." *Feedough,* July 8, 2021. https://www.feedough.com/history-of-whatsapp/.

"Paid Old Age Homes in Kottayam, Kerala: St. Mathews Home." 2021. St. Mathews' Home for Senior Citizens, 2021. https://www.mathewshome.org/.

Pandey, Kundan. 2020. "COVID-19 Lockdown Highlights India's Great Digital Divide." *DownToEarth,* July 20, 2020. https://www.downtoearth.org.in/news/governance/covid-19-lockdown-highlights-india-s-great-digital-divide-72514.

Parreñas, Rhacel Salazar. 2001. *Servants of Globalization: Women, Migration and Domestic Work.* Stanford, CA: Stanford University Press.

———. 2008. *The Force of Domesticity: Filipina Migrants and Globalization.* New York: NYU Press.

Pearce, Warren, Suay M. Özkula, Amanda K. Greene, Lauren Teeling, Jennifer S. Bansard, Janna Joceli Omena, and Elaine Teixeira Rabello. 2020. "Visual Cross-Platform Analysis: Digital Methods to Research Social Media Images." *Information, Communication and Society* 23 (2): 161–180. https://doi.org/10.1080/1369118X.2018.1486871.

Percot, Marie. 2006. "Indian Nurses in the Gulf: Two Generations of Female Migration." *South Asia Research* 26 (1): 41–62. https://doi.org/10.1177/0262728006063198.

———. 2012. "Transnational Masculinity: Indian Nurses' Husbands in Ireland." *e-Migrinter,* no. 8 (April): 74–86. https://doi.org/10.4000/e-migrinter.630.

———. 2014. "Un métier pour partir: La migration des infirmières kéralaises (Inde du Sud)." *Revue Tiers Monde* 217 (1): 45–59.

———. 2016. "Choosing a Profession in Order to Leave." In *South Asian Migration to Gulf Countries: History, Policies, Development,* edited by P. C. Jain and G. Z. Oommen, 247–263. London: Routledge.

Percot, Marie, and Sebastian Irudaya Rajan. 2007. "Female Emigration from India: Case Study of Nurses." *Economic and Political Weekly* 42 (4): 318–325.

Philip, Shaju. 2011. "Rapid Ageing Challenges Kerala." *Indian Express*, October 10, 2011. https://indianexpress.com/article/news-archive/web/rapid-ageing-challenges-kerala/.

Philips, Amali. 2003. "Stridhanam: Rethinking Dowry, Inheritance and Women's Resistance among the Syrian Christians of Kerala." *Anthropologica* 45 (2): 245–263. https://doi.org/10.2307/25606144.

———. 2004. "Gendering Colour: Identity, Femininity and Marriage in Kerala." *Anthropologica* 46 (2): 253–272. https://doi.org/10.2307/25606198.

Pink, Sarah, Heather Horst, John Postill, Larissa Hjorth, Tania Lewis, and Jo Tacchi. 2015. *Digital Ethnography: Principles and Practice*. London: SAGE.

Planning Commission of the Government of India. 2008. "Kerala Development Report." New Delhi: Academic Foundation.

Pols, Jeannette. 2005. "Enacting Appreciations: Beyond the Patient Perspective." *Health Care Analysis* 13 (3): 103–221. https://doi.org/10.1007/s10728-005-6448-6.

———. 2011. "Wonderful Webcams: About Active Gazes and Invisible Technologies." *Science, Technology, and Human Values* 36 (4): 451–473. https://doi.org/10.1177/0162243910366134.

———. 2012. *Care at a Distance: On the Closeness of Technology*. Amsterdam: Amsterdam University Press. https://library.oapen.org/viewer/web/viewer.html?file=/bitstream/handle/20.500.12657/34550/413032.pdf.

———. 2013. *De Chronificering van Het Ziek-Zijn: Empirische Ethiek in de Zorg = The Chronification of Illness: Empirical Ethics in Care*. Amsterdam: University of Amsterdam. https://hdl.handle.net/11245/1.515023.

———. 2014. "Radical Relationality: Epistemology in Care and Care Ethics for Research." In *Moral Boundaries Redrawn: The Significance of Joan Tronto's Argument for Political Theory, Professional Ethics, and Care as Practice*, edited by G. Olthuis, H. Kohlen, and J. Heier, 175–194. Leuven, the Netherlands: Peeters.

Pols, Jeannette, and Ingunn Moser. 2009. "Cold Technologies versus Warm Care? On Affective and Social Relations with and through Care Technologies." *ALTER-European Journal of Disability Research* 3 (2):159–178. https://doi.org/10.1016/j.alter.2009.01.003.

Prendergast, David, and Chiara Garattini. 2015. *Aging and the Digital Life Course*. New York: Berghahn.

Prescott, Megan, and Mark Nichter. 2014. "Transnational Nurse Migration: Future Directions for Medical Anthropological Research." *Social Science and Medicine* 107 (April): 113–123. https://doi.org/10.1016/j.socscimed.2014.02.026.

Pype, Katrien. 2018. "On Interference and Hotspots: Ethnographic Explorations of Rural-Urban Connectivity in and around Kinshasa's Phonie Cabins." *Mededelingen der Zittingen* 62 (2): 229–260.

Raghuram, Parvati. 2012. "Global Care, Local Configurations—Challenges to Conceptualizations of Care." *Global Networks* 12 (2): 155–174. https://doi.org/10.1111/j.1471-0374.2012.00345.x.

———. 2016. "Locating Care Ethics beyond the Global North." *ACME: An International Journal for Critical Geographies* 15 (3): 511–533.

Rajan, Sebastian Irudaya. 2002. "Home away from Home: A Survey of Old Age Homes and Inmates in Kerala, India." *Journal of Housing For the Elderly* 16 (1–2): 125–150. https://doi.org/10.1300/J081v16n01_09.

———, ed. 2022. *Handbook of Aging, Health and Public Policy: Perspectives from Asia*. Singapore: Springer.

Rajan, Sebastian Irudaya, and U. R. Arya. 2018. "Invisible Suffering of Elderly People Among Families in Kerala: Neglect and Abuse." In *Abuse and Neglect of the Elderly in India*, edited by Mala Kapur Shankardass and Sebastian Irudaya Rajan, 79–90. Singapore: Springer.

Rajan, Sebastian Irudaya, and Sanjay Kumar. 2003. "Living Arrangements among Indian Elderly: New Evidence from National Family Health Survey." *Economic and Political Weekly* 38 (1): 75–80. http://www.jstor.org/stable/4413048.

Rajan, Sebastian Irudaya, and Kunniparampil Curien Zachariah, eds. 2012. *Kerala's Demographic Future: Issues and Policy Options*. New Delhi: Academic Foundation.

———. 2019. "Emigration and Remittances: New Evidences from the Kerala Migration Survey 2018." Working Paper 483. Thiruvananthapuram, India: Centre for Development Studies. https://cds.edu/wp-content/uploads/WP483.pdf.

Raman, K. Ravi. 2010. *Development, Democracy and the State: Critiquing the Kerala Model of Development*. London: Routledge.

Ranjith, dir. 2013. *Kadal Kadannu Oru Mathukkutty*. India: Satyam Audios. DVD video.

Rao, Nivedita. 2018. "Who Is Paying for India's Healthcare?" *The Wire*, April 14, 2018. https://thewire.in/health/who-is-paying-for-indias-healthcare.

Rastogi, Mudita, and Karen S. Wampler. 1999. "Adult Daughters' Perceptions of the Mother–Daughter Relationship: A Cross-Cultural Comparison." *Family Relations* 48 (3): 327–336. https://doi.org/10.2307/585643.

Raval, Vaishali V., and Michael J. Kral. 2004. "Core versus Periphery: Dynamics of Personhood over the Life-Course for a Gujarati Hindu Woman." *Culture and Psychology* 10 (2): 162–194. https://doi.org/10.1177/1354067X04040927.

Ray, Panchali. 2019. *Politics of Precarity: Gendered Subjects and the Health Care Industry in Contemporary Kolkata*. New Delhi: Oxford University Press.

Ray, Raka, and Seemin Qayum. 2009. *Cultures of Servitude: Modernity, Domesticity, and Class in India*. Stanford, CA: Stanford University Press.

Reddy, Pushkar. 2018. "Do Historical Narratives Create Social Norms? The Case of Syrian Christians and Malabari Jews in Kerala." *Economic and Political Weekly* 53 (35). http://dspace.jgu.edu.in:8080/jspui/handle/10739/2512.

Reserve Bank of India. 2018. "India's Inward Remittances Survey 2016–17." Mumbai: RBI.

Riedel, Barbara. 2018. "Old and Emerging Cosmopolitan Traditions at the Malabar Coast of South India: A Study with Muslim Students in Kozhikode, Kerala." In *Beyond Cosmopolitanism: Towards Planetary Transformations*, edited by Ananta Kumar Giri, 257–274. Singapore: Springer. https://doi.org/10.1007/978-981-10-5376-4_14.

Risseeuw, Carla. 1991. *Gender Transformation, Power and Resistance among Women in Sri Lanka: The Fish Don't Talk about the Water*. New Delhi: Manohar.

Rodríguez-Muñiz, Michael. 2016. "Bridgework: STS, Sociology, and the 'Dark Matters' of Race." *Engaging Science, Technology, and Society* 2: 214–226. https://doi.org/10.17351/ests2016.74.

Roy, Adrija, Arvind Kumar Singh, Shree Mishra, Aravinda Chinnadurai, Arun Mitra, and Ojaswini Bakshi. 2020. "Mental Health Implications of COVID-19 Pandemic and Its Response in India." *International Journal of Social Psychiatry* 67 (5): 587–600. https://doi.org/10.1177/0020764020950769.

Roy, Arundhati. 2002. "God's Own Country." In *Where the Rain Is Born: Writings about Kerala*, edited by Anita Nair, 219–292. New Delhi: Penguin.

Rutten, Mario, and Pravin J. Patel. 2003. "Indian Migrants in Britain." *Asia Europe Journal* 1 (3): 403–417. https://doi.org/10.1007/s10308-003-0022-3.

Saikiran, K. P. 2020. "Kerala Government Staff's Salary Doubled in Last Seven Years." *Times of India*, June 20, 2020. https://timesofindia.indiatimes.com/city/thiruvananthapuram/kerala-government-staffs-salary-doubled-in-last-seven-years-report/articleshow/76477047.cms.

Salerno, Roger A. 2003. *Landscapes of Abandonment: Capitalism, Modernity, and Estrangement*. New York: SUNY Press.

Sampat, Kinjal, and Nandini Dey. 2017. "The Elderly in India's Informal Workforce Often Can't Retire, Even If They Want To." *Scroll.In*, April 21, 2017. https://scroll.in/article /835125/the-elderly-in-indias-informal-workforce-often-cant-retire-even-if-they-want-to.

Sax, William Sturman. 1991. *Mountain Goddess: Gender and Politics in a Himalayan Pilgrimage.* Oxford: Oxford University Press.

———. 2009. *God of Justice: Ritual Healing and Social Justice in the Central Himalayas.* Oxford: Oxford University Press.

Sebastian, Daliya, and T. V. Sekher. 2018. "Are Elderly People Safe in Their Own Households? New Evidence from Seven States of India." In *Abuse and Neglect of the Elderly in India,* 157–174. Singapore: Springer Nature.

Sebastian, Shevlin. 2020. "No One Cares for the Elderly." *KochiPost*, June 25, 2020. https:// kochipost.com/2020/06/25/no-one-cares-for-the-elderly/.

Selim, Jahangir, P.N.N. Nikhil, Ajay Bailey, and Anindita Datta. 2018. "Contextualizing Elder Abuse and Neglect in Institutional and Home Settings: Case Studies from India." In *Abuse and Neglect of the Elderly in India,* edited by Mala Kapur Shankardass and Sebastian Irudaya Rajan, 175–188. Boston: Springer.

Sengupta, Arghya. 2021. "The WhatsApp Nation." *Telegraph India*, February 20, 2021. https:// www.telegraphindia.com/opinion/the-whatsapp-nation-transaction-on-the-internet-is-a -faustian-bargain/cid/1804195.

Shankardass, Mala Kapur, and Sebastian Irudaya Rajan. 2018. *Abuse and Neglect of the Elderly in India.* Singapore: Springer Nature.

Simon, Elizabeth B. 2009. "Christianity and Nursing in India: A Remarkable Impact." *Journal of Christian Nursing* 26 (2): 88–94. https://doi.org/10.1097/01.CNJ.0000348266 .97429.6e.

Sørensen, Ninna Nyberg, and Ide Marie Vammen. 2014. "Who Cares? Transnational Families in Debates on Migration and Development." *New Diversities* 16 (2): 89–108.

Sprague, Sean. 2002. "Coconuts and Bishops: Ecumenical Advances from the Heart of India's Bible Belt." *One Magazine*, September–October 2002. https://cnewa.org/magazine /coconuts-and-bishops-30961/.

Srivastava, Dea. 2020. "#ItsBetweenYou: WhatsApp's First-Ever Brand Campaign!" *Do Your Thng*, August 5, 2020. https://blog.doyourthng.com/2020/08/05/itsbetweenyou-whatsapps -first-ever-brand-campaign/.

Summers, Charlotte. 2020. "Critical Care Beds Are No Use without Enough Specialist Staff." *The Guardian*, October 20, 2020. https://www.theguardian.com/commentisfree/2020 /oct/20/specialist-staff-critical-care-beds-winter-nhs-covid.

Sunny, Justin, Jajati K. Parida, and Mohammed Azurudeen. 2020. "Remittances, Investment and New Emigration Trends in Kerala." *Review of Development and Change* 25 (1): 5–29. https://doi.org/10.1177/0972266120932484.

Surendranath, Nidhi. 2014. "Increasing Number of Elderly Abandoned by Family." *The Hindu*, July 2, 2014. https://www.thehindu.com/todays-paper/tp-national/tp-kerala/increasing -number-of-elderly-abandoned-by-family/article6168438.ece.

Swiderski, Richard Michael. 1988. "Northists and Southists: A Folklore of Kerala Christians." *Asian Folklore Studies* 47 (1): 73–92. https://doi.org/10.2307/1178253.

Thomas. 2013. "Digital Literacy and IT Penetration in Kerala and Public Investments." *ZYXware Technologies*, August 11, 2013. https://www.zyxware.com/articles/3428/digital-literacy-and -it-penetration-in-kerala-and-public-investments.

Thomas, P. 2006. "The International Migration of Indian Nurses." *International Nursing Review* 53 (4): 277–283. https://doi.org/10.1111/j.1466-7657.2006.00494.x.

Thomas, Pradip Ninan. 2014. "Public Sector Software and the Revolution: Digital Literacy in Communist Kerala." *Media, Culture and Society* 36 (2): 258–268. https://doi.org/10.1177/0163443714526553.

Thomas, Sonja. 2016. "The Tying of the Ceremonial Wedding Thread: A Feminist Analysis of 'Ritual' and 'Tradition' Among Syro-Malabar Catholics in India." *Journal of Global Catholicism* 1 (1): 104–116. https://doi.org/10.32436/2475-6423.1008.

———. 2018. *Privileged Minorities: Syrian Christianity, Gender, and Minority Rights in Postcolonial India*. Seattle: University of Washington Press.

Timmons, Stephen, Catrin Evans, and Sreelekha Nair. 2016. "The Development of the Nursing Profession in a Globalised Context: A Qualitative Case Study in Kerala, India." *Social Science and Medicine* 166 (October): 41–48. https://doi.org/10.1016/j.socscimed.2016.08.012.

TNM Staff. 2018. "Kerala Nurses Call off Strike as Govt Issues Notification for Pay Revision." *The News Minute*, April 24, 2018. https://www.thenewsminute.com/article/kerala-nurses-call-strike-govt-issues-notification-pay-revision-80108.

Trawick, Margaret. 1990. *Notes on Love in a Tamil Family*. Berkeley: University of California Press.

Tronto, Joan. 1993. *Moral Boundaries: A Political Argument for an Ethic of Care*. London: Routledge.

UCA News Staff. 1989. "Kottayam in Kerala State Achieves 100 Percent Literacy in 100 Days." *Union of Catholic Asian News*, August 23, 1989. https://www.ucanews.com/story-archive/?post_name=/1989/08/24/kottayam-in-kerala-state-achieves-100-percent-literacy-in-100-days&post_id=38451.

United Nations. 1999. "Human Development Report." New York: UN.

———. 2013. "International Migration Report 2013." New York: UN.

———. 2017a. "International Migrant Stock: The 2017 Revision." New York: UN.

———. 2017b. "World Population Aging: 2017—Highlights." New York: UN.

Van Dullemen, Caroline E., and Jeanne G. M. de Bruijn. 2015. "Micro Pensions for Women; Initiatives and Challenges in India." *Ageing International* 40 (2): 98–116. https://doi.org/10.1007/s12126-014-9207-x.

Varma, Vishnu. 2021. "The Horrors of Kerala's Dowry Deaths." *Indian Express*, July 3, 2021. https://indianexpress.com/article/india/kerala/the-horrors-of-kerala-dowry-deaths-7387077/.

Vatuk, Sylvia. 1990. "'To Be a Burden on Others': Dependency Anxiety among the Elderly in India." In *Divine Passions: The Social Construction of Emotion in India*, edited by Owen M. Lynch, 64–88. Berkeley: University of California Press.

Vera-Sanso, Penny. 2006. "Experiences in Old Age: A South Indian Example of How Functional Age Is Socially Structured." *Oxford Development Studies* 34 (4): 457–472. https://doi.org/10.1080/13600810601045817.

Vertovec, Steven. 2004. "Cheap Calls: The Social Glue of Migrant Transnationalism." *Global Networks* 4 (2): 219–224. https://doi.org/10.1111/j.1471-0374.2004.00088.x.

Vishwanathan, Vivina. 2013. "What's the Real Cost of Retirement Homes?" *Mint*, August 27, 2013. https://www.livemint.com/Money/dvN4ue8SccGtABovRXLthI/Whats-the-real-cost-of-retirement-homes.html.

Visvanathan, Susan. 1989. "Marriage, Birth and Death: Property Rights and Domestic Relationships of the Orthodox/Jacobite Syrian Christians of Kerala." *Economic and Political Weekly* 24 (24): 1341–1346.

———. 1999. *The Christians of Kerala: History, Belief and Ritual among the Yakoba*. Delhi: Oxford Academic.

Voigt-Graf, Carmen. 2005. "The Construction of Transnational Spaces by Indian Migrants in Australia." *Journal of Ethnic and Migration Studies* 31 (2): 365–384. https://doi.org/10.1080/1369183042000339972.

Von Faber, Margaret, and Sjaak van der Geest. 2010. "Losing and Gaining: About Growing Old 'Successfully' in the Netherlands." In *Contesting Aging and Loss*, edited by Janice E. Graham and Peter H. Stephenson, 27–45. Toronto: University of Toronto Press.

Vora, Neha. 2013. *Impossible Citizens: Dubai's Indian Diaspora*. Durham, NC: Duke University Press.

Wadhwa, Soma. 2004. "And He Can Keep It." *Outlook*, July 12, 2004. https://india.eu.org/spip.php?article1993.

Wajcman, Judy. 2016. *Pressed for Time: The Acceleration of Life in Digital Capitalism*. London: University of Chicago Press.

Walton-Roberts, Margaret. 2010. "Student Nurses and Their Post Graduation Migration Plans: A Kerala Case Study." In *India Migration Report 2010*, edited by Sebastian Irudaya Rajan, 196–216. London: Routledge.

———. 2012. "Contextualizing the Global Nursing Care Chain: International Migration and the Status of Nursing in Kerala, India." *Global Networks* 12 (2): 175–194. https://doi.org/10.1111/j.1471-0374.2012.00346.x.

Walton-Roberts, Margaret, Vivien Runnels, S. Irudaya Rajan, Atul Sood, Sreelekha Nair, Philomina Thomas, Corinne Packer, et al. 2017. "Causes, Consequences, and Policy Responses to the Migration of Health Workers: Key Findings from India." *Human Resources for Health* 15 (1): 28. https://doi.org/10.1186/s12960-017-0199-y.

The Week Staff. 2020. "Kerala Leads the Way, Again: Mosque Set to Host Hindu Wedding." April 1, 2020. https://www.theweek.in/news/india/2020/01/04/kerala-leads-the-way-again-mosque-set-to-host-hindu-wedding.html.

Wilding, Raelene. 2006. "'Virtual' Intimacies? Families Communicating across Transnational Contexts." *Global Networks* 6 (2): 125–142. https://doi.org/10.1111/j.1471-0374.2006.00137.x.

Willems, Dick, and Jeannette Pols. 2010. "Goodness! The Empirical Turn in Health Care Ethics." *Medische Antropologie* 22 (1): 161–170.

Winance, Myriam. 2007. "Being Normally Different? Changes to Normalization Processes: From Alignment to Work on the Norm." *Disability and Society* 22 (6): 625–638. https://doi.org/10.1080/09687590701560261.

———. 2010. "Care and Disability: Practices of Experimenting, Tinkering with, and Arranging People and Technical Aids." In *Care in Practice. On Tinkering in Clinics, Homes and Farms*, edited by Annemarie Mol, Ingunn Moser, and Jeannette Pols, 93–117. Bielefeld, Germany: Transcript Verlag.

World Health Organization. 2012. "Connecting and Caring: Innovations for Healthy Ageing." *Bulletin of the World Health Organization* 90 (3): 157–244.

Xu, Wenqian. 2020. "(Non-)Stereotypical Representations of Older People in Swedish Authority-Managed Social Media." *Ageing and Society* 42 (3): 719–740. https://doi.org/10.1017/S0144686X20001075.

Yates-Doerr, Emily. 2017. "Where Is the Local?: Partial Biologies, Ethnographic Sitings." *HAU: Journal of Ethnographic Theory* 7 (2): 377–401. https://doi.org/10.14318/hau7.2.032.

———. 2019. "Whose Global, Which Health? Unsettling Collaboration with Careful Equivocation." *American Anthropologist* 121 (2): 297–310. https://doi.org/10.1111/aman.13259.

Yates-Doerr, Emily, and Megan A. Carney. 2016. "Demedicalizing Health: The Kitchen as a Site of Care." *Medical Anthropology* 35 (4): 305–321.

Yeates, Nicola. 2009. *Globalizing Care Economies and Migrant Workers: Explorations in Global Care Chains*. New York: Palgrave Macmillan.

————. 2012. "Global Care Chains: A State-of-the-Art Review and Future Directions in Care Transnationalization Research." *Global Networks* 12 (2): 135–154. https://doi.org/10.1111/j .1471-0374.2012.00344.x.

Yeoh, Brenda S. A., and Kamalini Ramdas. 2014. "Gender, Migration, Mobility and Transnationalism." *Gender, Place and Culture* 21 (10): 1197–1213. https://doi.org/10.1080/0966369X .2014.969686.

Yousuf, Kabeer. 2020. "TRA Lifts Ban on VoIP Calls." *Oman Daily Observer*, March 17, 2020. https://www.omanobserver.om/article/14684/Head stories/tra-lifts-ban-on-voip-calls.

Zachariah, Kunniparampil Curien, Elangikal Thomas Mathew, and Sebastian Irudaya Rajan. 2003. *Dynamics of Migration in Kerala: Dimensions, Differentials, and Consequences.* New Delhi: Orient Blackswan.

Zachariah, Kunniparampil Curien, and Sebastian Irudaya Rajan. 2015. *Dynamics of Emigration and Remittances in Kerala: Results from the Kerala Migration Survey 2014.* Thiruvananthapuram, India: Centre for Development Studies.

INDEX

Note: Page numbers in *italics* indicate figures.

ABOUT THE AUTHOR

TANJA AHLIN finished her PhD at the University of Amsterdam, where she has since worked as a lecturer and postdoctoral researcher. Her academic publications include a number of articles and book chapters on technology, care, aging, migration, gender, and methods. Among other books, she has translated a collection of poetry by Mary Oliver into Slovenian.

Available titles in the Medical Anthropology:
Health, Inequality, and Social Justice series

Carina Heckert, *Fault Lines of Care: Gender, HIV, and Global Health in Bolivia*

Joel Christian Reed, *Landscapes of Activism: Civil Society and HIV and AIDS Care in Northern Mozambique*

Alison Heller, *Fistula Politics: Birthing Injuries and the Quest for Continence in Niger*

Jessica Hardin, *Faith and the Pursuit of Health: Cardiometabolic Disorders in Samoa*

Beatriz M. Reyes-Foster, *Psychiatric Encounters: Madness and Modernity in Yucatan, Mexico*

Sonja van Wichelen, *Legitimating Life: Adoption in the Age of Globalization and Biotechnology*

Andrea Whittaker, *International Surrogacy as Disruptive Industry in Southeast Asia*

Lesley Jo Weaver, *Sugar and Tension: Diabetes and Gender in Modern India*

Ellen Block and Will McGrath, *Infected Kin: Orphan Care and AIDS in Lesotho*

Nolan Kline, *Pathogenic Policing: Immigration Enforcement and Health in the U.S. South*

Ciara Kierans, *Chronic Failures: Kidneys, Regimes of Care, and the Mexican State*

Stéphanie Larchanché, *Cultural Anxieties: Managing Migrant Suffering in France*

Dvera I. Saxton, *The Devil's Fruit: Farmworkers, Health, and Environmental Justice*

Siri Suh, *Dying to Count: Post-Abortion Care and Global Reproductive Health Politics in Senegal*

Vania Smith-Oka, *Becoming Gods: Medical Training in Mexican Hospitals*

Daria Trentini, *At Ansha's: Life in the Spirit Mosque of a Healer in Mozambique*

Mette N. Svendsen, *Near Human: Border Zones of Species, Life, and Belonging*

Cristina A. Pop, *The Cancer Within: Reproduction, Cultural Transformation, and Health Care in Romania*

Elizabeth J. Pfeiffer, *Viral Frictions: Global Health and the Persistence of HIV Stigma in Kenya*

Anna Versfeld, *Making Uncertainty: Tuberculosis, Substance Use, and Pathways to Health in South Africa*

Tanja Ahlin, *Calling Family: Digital Technologies and the Making of Transnational Care Collectives*